D1623099

eDiets.com®:
A Decade of Life-Changing Success

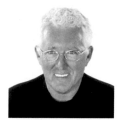

David R. Humble
Founder/CEO, eDiets.com

Breaking New Ground

Dave Humble likes to think outside the box. So in 1996, when he thought about leveraging the power of the Internet to bring diet and fitness solutions to everyone, it seemed like a great idea. His new company, eDiets.com, ushered in a new era of convenient online dieting.

A Decade of Diet Success

eDiets has remained at the forefront of the industry. With a history of ground-breaking industry "firsts," more than two million members, and international programs in the United Kingdom, Germany and Spain, eDiets.com has become the Internet's leading diet and fitness destination.

eDiets Weight Loss Solutions

This comprehensive weight-loss resource has been published in partnership with Time Inc. Home Entertainment in celebration of eDiets' 10th anniversary. It provides essential information for anyone who wants to lose or maintain weight, exercise more effectively or improve overall health.

We hope that you will find these solutions helpful in your personal weight-loss journey.

#1 Health, Fitness & Nutrition Site 2004
— Nielsen//NetRatings

"Best of the Web" & "Forbes Favorite"
2002, 2004 & 2005
— Forbes.com

Editors' Choice 2004 & 2005
— *PC Magazine*

"Excellent!"
— as recommended on NBC's *TODAY Show*

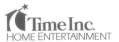

Publisher: Richard Fraiman
Executive Director, Marketing Services: Carol Pittard
Director, Retail & Special Sales: Tom Mifsud
Marketing Director, Branded Businesses: Swati Rao
Director, New Product Development: Peter Harper
Financial Director: Steven Sandonato
Prepress Manager: Emily Rabin
Book Production Manager: Jonathan Polsky
Product Manager: Victoria Alfonso
Associate Prepress Manager: Anne-Michelle Gallero

Special thanks:
Bozena Bannett, Glenn Buonocore, Suzanne Janso, Robert Marasco, Brooke McGuire, Chavaughn Raines,
Ilene Schreider, Adriana Tierno, Britney Williams

Copyright 2006
Time Inc. Home Entertainment

Published by Time Inc. Home Entertainment
Time Inc.
1271 Avenue of the Americas
New York, New York 10020

All rights reserved. No part of this book may be reproduced in any form or by any electronic or mechanical means, including information storage and retrieval systems, without permission in writing from the publisher, except by a reviewer, who may quote brief passages in a review.

ISBN: 1-933405-11-2

Printed in China

Time Inc. Home Entertainment is a trademark of Time Inc.

We welcome your comments and suggestions about eDiets Weight Loss Solutions. Please write to us at:
eDiets - Attention: TIHE Book Editors - PO Box 11016 - Des Moines, IA 50336-1016

If you would like to order any of our hardcover Collector's Edition books, please call us at 1-800-327-6388.
(Monday through Friday, 7:00 a.m.— 8:00 p.m. or Saturday, 7:00 a.m.— 6:00 p.m. Central Time).

eDiets.com
Find your perfect diet!

Editor-in-Chief:
John McGran

Managing Editors:
Nel Hernandez & Lori Savka

Senior Editor:
Vanessa Rush

Contributing Editors:
Kim Droze, Glenn Mueller & Che Odom

Creative Director:
Lori Savka

Art Directors:
David Kopet, Beni Mendez & Rodrigo Minozzi

Designers:
Paul Ho-On & Jefferson Junatas

Photo Credits:
Glamour Shots, Nino Rakichevich Photography, Richard Anderson (Anderson Photo Graphics), Getty Images, ShutterStock and FotoSearch

Contributors:
Lesa Amy, MS, RD, LD/N
Dr. Matthew Anderson, D. Min.
Kandee Biren, LMHC
Susan Burke, MS, RD, LD/N, CDE
Raphael Calzadilla, BA, CPT, ACE
Ellen DeLalla, RN, LMHC
Carolina Diaz-Bordon
Julia Griggs Havey
Jason Knapfel
Dr. Susan Mendelsohn, Psy.D.
Christine E. Miller, MS, RD, LD/N, CDE
Pamela Ofstein, MS, RD, LD/N
Dr. John Sklare, Ed.D.
Dr. Nancy Tice, D.O.

Special thanks:
Bob Greene, BFA, MFA & Bill Phillips

eDiets and eDiets.com are registered trademarks of eDiets.com, Inc. 3801 W. Hillsboro Blvd., Deerfield Beach, FL 33442

Visit us online at www.eDiets.com.

CONTENTS

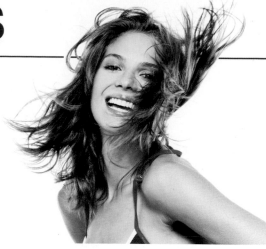

■ INTRODUCTION

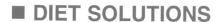

■ DIET SOLUTIONS

CONTENTS

■ FITNESS SOLUTIONS

■ MOTIVATION SOLUTIONS

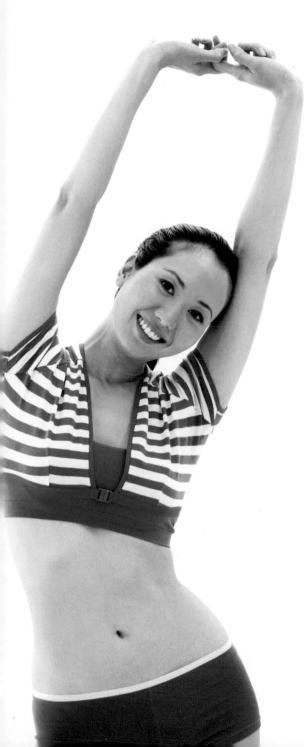

■ NUTRITION TOOLS

■ PROGRESS JOURNAL

■ REAL PEOPLE, REAL RESULTS

Look for real-life stories of dieting success throughout *eDiets Weight Loss Solutions*. Whether you have a little or a lot to lose, you're bound to share the challenges that these successful dieters faced. Get inspired!

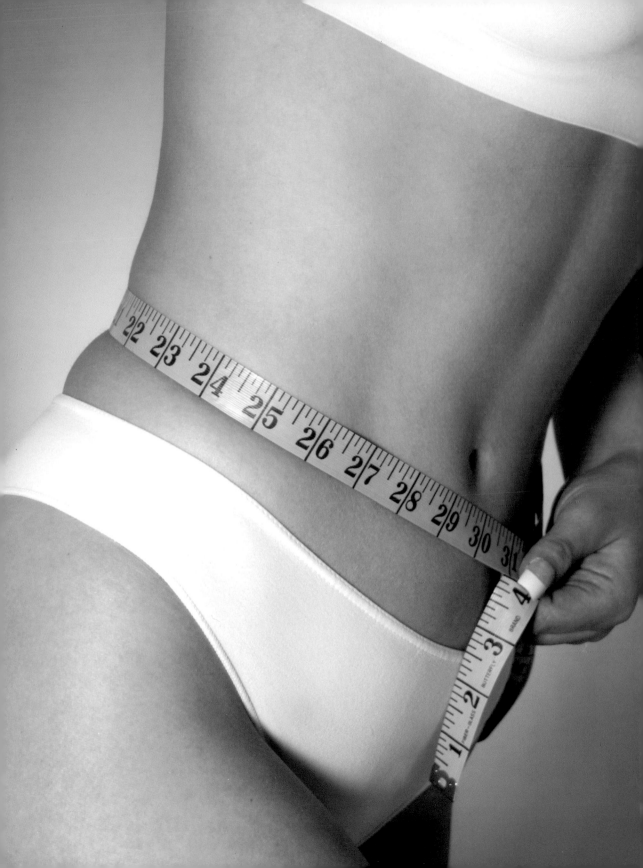

Do You Need to
Lose Weight?

America is facing an obesity epidemic. If you live in the United States, chances are you or others you know are overweight. If you find that difficult to believe, just take a look around you. Super-sized meals have created super-sized waistlines for a growing number of Americans ... including children. And those numbers are rising fast.

If you're thinking about losing weight, your first step is to set a goal and several reasonable milestones. Start by determining your healthy goal weight. **The Body Mass Index** (BMI) is the medical standard for determining a person's healthy weight. It identifies a healthy weight range for men and women based on their height and weight. Use the BMI chart on Page 8 to find your healthy weight and to help you set your weight-loss goal.

▷ Why Are You Overweight?

Next, look at the real reasons you've gained weight. Yes, food is a big part of the equation. But WHY you eat and WHEN you eat are just as important as WHAT you eat. Start by identifying your problem eating behaviors, then take the necessary steps to change them.

- **Have you been overweight most of your life, or is your weight gain a recent problem?**
- **Do you eat when you're nervous or upset?**
- **Does food make you happy?**
- **Do you reward yourself with food?**
- **Do you constantly think about your weight?**
- **Are you a frequent snacker?**
- **Do you plan your meals in advance?**
- **Are you addicted to carbs?**

Answers to questions like these will give you a better understanding of your unhealthy eating behaviors.

The Changing Shape of America

More than 2/3 of American adults are overweight.
— *Time magazine, June 2004*

In the past 20 years, the average dress size of the American woman has gone from a size 8 to a size 14.
— *U.S. Centers for Disease Control and Prevention*

30% of American children are overweight or on their way to becoming overweight.
— *USA Today, June 4, 2004*

71 million Americans are currently on a diet.
— *Calorie Control Council Study, 2004*

More than 95% of people who begin a weight-loss program each year regain their pre-diet weight – or put on more pounds.
— *Federal Trade Commission, 2005*

Body Mass Index (BMI)

Body Mass Index (BMI) is a measure of body fat based on height and weight.

HOW TO FIND YOUR BMI:

1 - Find your height in the orange bar. Follow it over to your current weight.
2 - Follow your weight column up vertically to find your BMI in the red bar at the top of the chart.

Underweight = Less than 18.5
Normal Weight = 18.5-24.9

Overweight = 25-29.9
Obese = Greater than 30

BMI	19	20	21	22	23	24	25	26	27	28	29	30	31	32	33	34
Height							Body Weight (pounds)									
58"	91	96	100	105	110	115	119	124	129	134	138	143	148	153	158	162
59"	94	99	104	109	114	119	124	128	133	138	143	148	153	158	163	168
60"	97	102	107	112	118	123	128	133	138	143	148	153	158	163	168	174
61"	100	106	111	116	122	127	132	137	143	148	153	158	164	169	174	180
62"	104	109	115	120	126	131	136	142	147	153	158	164	169	175	180	186
63"	107	113	118	124	130	135	141	146	152	158	163	169	175	180	186	191
64"	110	116	122	128	134	140	145	151	157	163	169	174	180	186	192	197
65"	114	120	126	132	138	144	150	156	162	168	174	180	186	192	198	204
66"	118	124	130	136	142	148	155	161	167	173	179	186	192	198	204	210
67"	121	127	134	140	146	153	159	166	172	178	185	191	198	204	211	217
68"	125	131	138	144	151	158	164	171	177	184	190	197	203	210	216	223
69"	128	135	142	149	155	162	169	176	182	189	196	203	209	216	223	230
70"	132	139	146	153	160	167	174	181	188	195	202	209	216	222	229	236
71"	136	143	150	157	165	172	179	186	193	200	208	215	222	229	236	243
72"	140	147	154	162	169	177	184	191	199	206	213	221	228	235	242	250
73"	144	151	159	166	174	182	189	197	204	212	219	227	235	242	250	257
74"	148	155	163	171	179	186	194	202	210	218	225	233	241	249	256	264
75"	152	160	168	176	184	192	200	208	216	224	232	240	248	256	264	272
76"	156	164	172	180	189	197	205	213	221	230	238	246	254	263	271	279

Healthy Weight Range   Overweight Range

www.eDiets.com

Once you've identified your problem eating behaviors, you'll need a plan to change them. Developing healthy new habits to replace the unhealthy ones is the key to long-term success. If you don't change the underlying behavior problems, you may lose the weight, but you will likely gain it back when you stop dieting and return to your "normal" way of eating.

A good lifestyle assessment tool like the **eDiets® Diet Needs Analysis**™ can help you identify the habits and behaviors that have contributed to your weight gain. It can also identify the best all-around programs to help you take control of your weight. (To take the free Diet Needs Analysis, visit **www.eDiets.com/dna.**)

▷ What Do You Need to Succeed?

THE BIG 3: DIET, FITNESS & MOTIVATION

Once you've found your healthy weight range on the BMI chart, established your personal weight-loss goal and identified your eating behaviors, you'll need to develop a winning game plan to help you reach your goal. Your plan should have three key components:

- **A diet that you can easily follow that fits your lifestyle**
- **A workout plan designed for your fitness level**
- **Motivation boosters and behavior modification techniques**

On the following pages, you will find a wealth of important information to help you formulate your personal weight-management plan. The **Diet Solutions** section offers an overview of popular weight-loss plans, a variety of healthy dieting tips, delicious healthy recipes and much more. In the **Fitness Solutions** section, we'll share spot exercises that target specific body parts and workout tips from celebrity fitness trainer, Bob Greene. The third section, **Motivation Solutions**, offers expert insight into motivation, behavior modification and more. Together, these three solutions will provide you with the tools you need to help you build your own personal success plan. Then, use the **Nutrition Tools** in section four and the **Progress Journal** in section five to help keep you on track everyday.

Here's to a healthy new you!
The eDiets Expert Team

Diet
SOLUTIONS

Changing unhealthy eating behaviors can be easier when you choose the right weight-loss plan. Follow these dieting dos and don'ts on your journey to a healthy new you.

What's Your
Dieting Style?

If you're ready to start a weight-loss program, start by finding a method that will work for you. You can follow a diet book, diet online, drive to diet meetings or buddy up with a friend. There are plenty of options out there, so choose the one that best fits your lifestyle and your needs.

▷ Online Dieting

The Internet has the potential to revolutionize the way America deals with its rising obesity epidemic. Using the Internet for weight loss lets you personalize a diet plan to fit your needs. And it's very convenient.

Internet dieting has exploded in the last few years, and it's easy to understand why. Web-based dieting is convenient and private. You can log on anywhere, anytime to get the information and support you need. It's affordable, and it's been proven effective.

A study conducted by the University of Vermont's Behavioral Weight Control Research Program found online dieting just as effective as offline programs in maintaining weight loss. And a study by researchers at the Brown University Medical School published in the *Journal of the American Medical Association* shows Internet-based weight-loss programs can help people lose weight. If you're looking for a convenient and supportive method, online dieting is it.

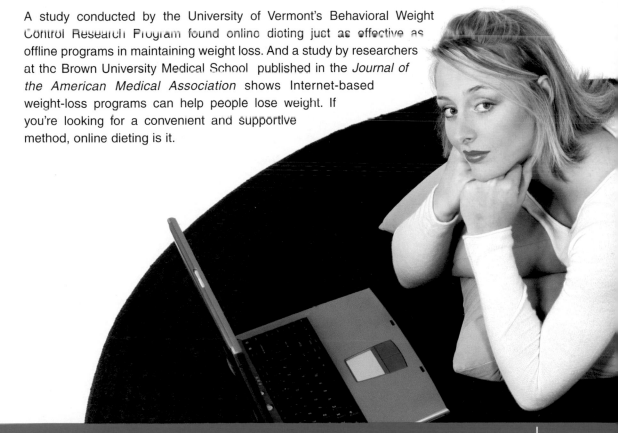

▷ Dieting by the Book

With several diet books on the New York Times® Bestseller list at any given time, you'll have lots of choices. But do your homework before you choose a plan. Find out how the diet works and what you can eat. Following a diet book can be effective with self-discipline and willpower.

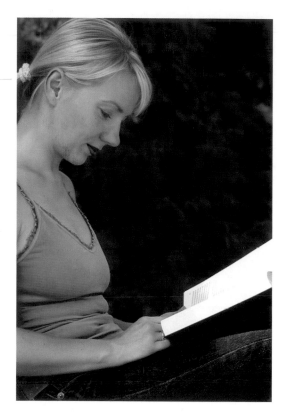

▷ Fancy Meeting You Here

Some diet programs hold weekly support meetings. While stepping on the scale in public may be daunting, the benefits may be worth it. At a drive-to meeting, you weigh in and take part in a discussion. Plans vary – there could be prescribed meal plans, a points system or other program features. Interacting with other dieters face-to-face can help keep you on track.

▷ Take a Diet Vacation

If you need a getaway and you're packing extra pounds, a weight-loss vacation might be right for you. For adults, luxurious services are available in posh settings. Attractive amenities are partnered with expert-conducted workshops and seminars that cover wellness topics. Most resorts are located in picturesque areas, so a focus on outdoor fitness is included. Weight-loss spas include food, of course, but the quality and quantity can vary greatly. Some may drastically limit calories, and a one-week stay can be expensive. Weight loss can also vary; some plans promise 1 to 2 pounds per day, and some promise even more. Safe, long-term weight loss is achieved when you drop the weight slowly – about two pounds per week is ideal.

For overweight children, the most reputable camps focus on wellness, nutrition and most of all, fun. Gone are the dreaded "fat camps"– kids these days are embarking on outdoor adventures, and it just so happens that they lose weight in the process. Support is key at these camps; knowledgeable, sympathetic counselors are integral to kids' success. A good camp will address the emotions of being an overweight child – depression, teasing, frustration – and help the child deal with those feelings. But for long-term weight loss, kids must learn healthy habits that they can continue following when they get home. Camps that focus on nutrition and healthy choices are the ones that help kids succeed in their weight-loss quest.

▷ Playing One-on-One

It makes sense to consult an expert before embarking on a diet plan – a dietitian or other nutrition expert can help assess your nutritional needs and choose the right diet for your lifestyle. Just make sure you check their credentials. While it can be pricey, a one-on-one approach provides privacy and more personal attention.

When it comes to incorporating fitness into a healthy lifestyle, the advice and instruction of a personal trainer is ideal for learning proper form, efficiency and injury prevention. It also makes working out at a gym less intimidating when you understand the proper use of equipment. The best trainers are certified by the American Council on Exercise.

▷ The Food Is in the Mail

For time-challenged dieters, a great strategy is having balanced meals and snacks delivered right to your door. Or, if your plan provides local offices that stock their foods, you can pick it up yourself. Having the right foods available when hunger strikes prevents bingeing on unfavorable choices, like sweets. Pre-portioned foods also eliminate calorie-, point- and carb-counting, making it easier to stay on track. Variety may be limited, but you may find a few favorites that become part of your regular menu. And, although more costly than recipe-based plans, the convenience and portion control are worth the price for many dieters.

Think about your lifestyle and the level of guidance and support you need. Then, choose the diet style that's right for you.

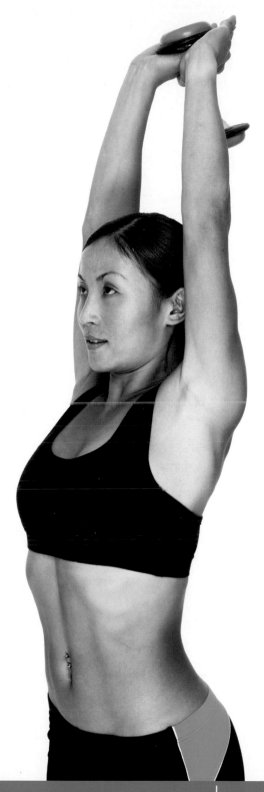

Challenge: Busy, on-the-go lifestyle	Start Weight: 130 lbs. End Weight: 109 lbs. Pounds Lost: 21

Results not typical.

Kerry Shares Her Secrets

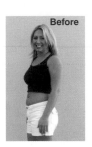
Before

Curvy Kerry P. loves the beach. She yearned for the day she could slip into an itsy-bitsy, teeny-weeny bikini and confidently stroll down the beach. Thin most of her life, Kerry watched her body expand as a result of too many fast-food lunches, late-night pizza runs and a lack of exercise.

At 130 pounds, she was miserable. Yes, 130 pounds doesn't sound so bad, but on Kerry's 5-foot 1-inch frame, the extra weight was enough to make her uncomfortable — especially because she works in the weight-loss industry.

"I saw someone I used to work with, and they asked if I just had a baby," she recalls. "Another acquaintance of mine hit me in the stomach and asked what was going on."

As an eDiets employee, dieting was constantly on her mind. She knew she would need a plan that would suit her busy lifestyle. That plan proved to be the Glycemic Impact Diet. In just five months, she made the amazing transformation from flab to fab. Today, she's maintaining her 21-pound loss at 109 pounds.

Before she got started, she consulted with

eDiets' Chief Fitness Pro, Raphael Calzadilla.

"Raphael told me I needed to eat more frequently throughout the day. I wanted something that was balanced and simple at the same time. I wanted to eat more healthful food."

Kerry used eDiets menus to plan her meals ahead of time. She cut down on salt and butter, which wasn't easy, and cut back on diet sodas, drinking just two a day. She also drank more water. After a couple of weeks, she noticed that she had more energy.

Kerry joined a gym and went a minimum of three times a week. She did 30 minutes of cardio exercise, built up to 45 minutes and incorporated strength training. Two months into her program, she began running regularly. Then she experimented with martial arts, beach volleyball and other activities.

Kerry soon began noticing marked improvements in endurance and strength.

"I feel a lot more confident and a lot happier; I can focus on other things. I realize that I really like doing physical activities and playing sports." These days, her focus is on maintaining her weight. She continues to follow a balanced meal plan and stays active.

Real People, Real Results.

Challenge:
Needed privacy and support

Start Weight: 149 lbs.
End Weight: 119 lbs.
Pounds Lost: 30

Results not typical.

Katie Needed Super Support

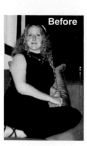
Before

Before Katie B. joined eDiets, she considered going to other programs where they had in-person meetings, but she felt uncomfortable and out of place. She couldn't relate to other dieters in the program who had different weight-loss approaches and goals.

"Maybe I didn't have as much weight to lose, or maybe I had more weight to lose than other people. I felt embarrassed about going in and sitting with other people who saw who I was," Katie says.

The anonymity of an online weight-loss program appealed to Katie because she says, "No one knew how much weight I had to lose or where I was in my weight-loss journey."

eDiets.com offers more than 100 support groups. This is the place to get expert and member support and assistance. It's a great way to build a terrific support network, too. In addition to the regular Support Groups, Katie found the challenge groups. It's highly recommended to join a challenge. These motivated Katie and kept her on track.

Katie particularly enjoyed the challenge group that she joined, the Castaweigh Challenge. It appealed to her because her team members had similar goals and concerns. There are groups for people trying to lose just a little weight and groups for those trying to lose 100 pounds or more. Katie says, "It was a perfect way for me to see where others might be in the journey, where I might be going and maybe help me predict any challenges I might face down the road."

Katie has been part of the challenge for more than two years, and it was the key to kick-starting her weight loss and keeping her motivated. The support and help Katie received from her team members kept Katie on plan, and she made some great friends in the process.

Katie now runs her team. "I don't feel complete if I don't go online every day and talk to them. I made some of the best friends in my life in my challenge group."

Finding the
Right Diet for You

With so many different diets to choose from, it can be difficult to tell which plan is right for you. Some diets cut carbs; others reduce fat. Some plans let you eat several times a day, while others limit you to three meals. In spite of all their differences, all diets have one thing in common – they can only help you lose weight if you reduce your daily calories.

Most diets work if you can commit yourself, but not all diets are created equal. The best diet for you is a diet you'd feel comfortable following for life. It has foods you like to eat, and it fits your lifestyle and your "natural" way of eating. It will help you lose weight and then, with some modification, it will help you keep it off.

▷ Map Your Course

The dieting journey is like a road trip. When you prepare for a road trip, you get a map to plan the route to your destination of choice. Then you just stay on course until you get there. When you go on a diet, the same principle holds true. You need a plan that will show you how to limit calories and change eating behavior. Find the right road map and follow it until you get there.

For most people, just "cutting back" on their usual diet isn't enough. A structured program helps change bad habits. It teaches you to eat the right foods and to identify proper portions.

▷ Go for Sustenance

Weight loss shouldn't be about deprivation. You may be able to do it for awhile, but ultimately, it will feel restrictive and unsatisfying, which may

lead to cheating. You don't have to eliminate the foods you love to lose weight. So choose a plan with the kind of foods you enjoy.

It is also important to avoid diets that are very low in calories. Most women need a minimum of 1,200 calories just to cover basic metabolic functions. Men need at least 1,500 calories. Low-calorie diets may produce quick weight loss, but experts say the quicker you lose the weight, the faster you put it back on.

Most diets work if you can commit yourself, but not all diets are created equal.

▷ One Is a Lonely Number

Dieting can be tough, so why go it alone? Get a little help from your friends by enlisting a diet or workout buddy, or get expert advice from a dietitian or personal trainer. This support will help you stay on track and achieve your weight-loss goal. The members of a support network can achieve more together than any of them would be able to accomplish on their own, according to Timothy Patton, a professor of public health at Florida International University.

▷ Stay Away from Fads

Avoid programs that are based on unscientific recommendations, like not eating fruits at the same time as proteins. Be wary of plans that include supplements. Although there are dozens of products out there that claim to burn

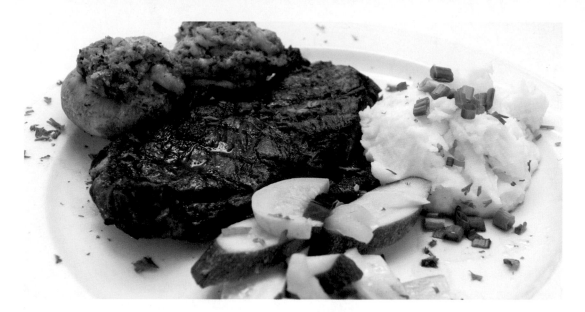

fat and build muscle, their benefits are often not what they assert, and they will not teach you how to eat healthfully.

Take a multivitamin every day. When you're restricting calories to lose weight, it's a quick and easy way to get the nutrients you need to stay healthy.

▷ Customize Your Plan

Choose a plan that fits the way you live. Don't choose a recipe-based plan if you don't have time to cook. A convenience plan that includes prepackaged foods like cereals, yogurt and frozen entrees may be a better choice. These can be balanced, nutritious foods that don't require a lot of planning or preparation.

Go for variety. When you get bored with eating the same foods, you lose motivation. So choose a balanced meal plan that's big on variety. High-fiber vegetables, whole grains, lean protein and healthy, monounsaturated fat from olive oil and fatty fish are the key ingredients of a healthy diet that you can live with – and lose with.

Eat on your body's natural schedule. Eating patterns are important. Do you like to eat just three meals a day? Or do you find that you get hungry in between meals? If so, eating smaller meals throughout the day might be a better plan.

Find a program that you can stick with for life. The best program becomes a maintenance program once you reach your goal weight. Find a plan you enjoy, then make it a habit. Once you reach your goal weight, stay with a maintenance version of the program you used to get there, at least for a full year. That's the surest way to keep the weight off. Modify your diet to add variety, then set your plan to "cruise control." Before you know it, you'll have a healthy new lifestyle.

▷ Your Bottom Line

When choosing a diet plan, budget is important. Normally, the most flexible and affordable plans are recipe-based. Look for foods that are on sale or buy ingredients in bulk to save money. Prepared foods offer the ultimate in dieting convenience. They will cost you more, but for the time-challenged dieter with no time to cook, weigh and measure, the convenience is well worth the price. Follow these tips to pinch pennies at the grocery store:

☑ **Stock up** — Buy large packages of meat, chicken and fish and wrap into smaller-sized portions to freeze. Less tender cuts of meat are cheaper and just as nutritious. Frozen is less expensive than fresh and just as nutritious. Eggs are inexpensive, so stock up if they're on your plan.

☑ **Manage your meal plan** — Economize by making more than two or three meals and recipes. You save on price when you buy in bulk and can freeze the remaining portions for your own convenience meals.

☑ **Cut and chop** — Premixed and washed salads and cut-up vegetables and fruit are convenient, but more expensive. Buy a head of lettuce, rinse it thoroughly then wrap in paper towels and store in a plastic bag in the refrigerator.

☑ **Buy on sale** — If your meal plan calls for blueberries and strawberries and they're in season, buy the large size. Rinse, pat dry, slice and freeze some. Use the rest as your fruit for the week.

☑ **Be flexible** — If your menu calls for steak and your budget calls for chicken, then substitute chicken or any other protein that's on sale, including fish or tofu.

☑ **Stick with water** — Water is the ultimate budget-friendly diet drink. But bottled water can be pricey; you can purchase a refrigerator water filter or under-the-sink model for less than $30, and it will save you money in the long run.

☑ **Save money on vegetables and fruit** — Buy in season and check the frozen food aisle for sales on frozen vegetables and fruit. Frozen produce, picked and processed in the field, retains more valuable nutrition than fresh produce. Local produce will be less expensive than shipped and is generally fresher.

☑ **Eat out economically** — Save money by sharing an entrée and ordering a salad for an appetizer. Dining out is usually more expensive than cooking at home, but an occasional night out can be made more economical by sharing. If you're dining alone, have the server wrap up half of your entrée and make it into two meals.

How to Choose a Diet

1. **Don't deprive yourself.**
   Choose a plan with the kind of foods you enjoy, or ultimately, you'll find the diet restrictive and unsatisfying.

2. **Avoid diets that are very low in calories.**
   The quicker you lose the weight, the quicker you'll put it back on. Drop the weight slowly – about 2 pounds per week.

3. **Stay away from fads.** Enough said.

4. **Eat on your body's natural schedule.**
   Do you like to eat three meals a day, or do you prefer smaller meals throughout the day?

5. **Choose a plan that fits the way you live.**
   If you don't want to cook, choose a flexible plan that includes convenience foods.

6. **Go for variety.**
   When you get bored with eating the same foods, you lose motivation.

7. **Remember your bottom line.**
   Budget is important. The most flexible and affordable plans are recipe-based. Convenience costs more, but for time-challenged dieters it's well worth the price.

8. **Get essential vitamins.**
   Take a multivitamin every day.

9. **Get a little help from your friends.**
   Dieting can be tough. So why go it alone? Reach out to a friend, or get expert advice.

10. **Do it for life.**
    The best program becomes a maintenance program once you reach your goal weight. Find a plan you enjoy, then make it a habit.

Understanding
Nutrition Labels

Nutrition labels can be confusing, but they contain the essential information you need to choose healthy foods. Nutrition labels are mandated and regulated by the FDA, and the required listings of ingredients often change. Familiarizing yourself with nutrition facts will help you make the right decisions. The chart below shows you how to read nutrition labels.

Read the serving size and total servings per package. Compare serving size to the amount you actually eat. Portion size matters, even with healthy foods.

% Daily values show how much of the daily recommended amounts of a nutrient is in a serving. *(Tip: 5% or less is considered low, and 20% DV or more is considered high for all nutrients.)*

A "free" food contains no (or just a trace of) fat, saturated fat, cholesterol, sodium, sugar and calories.

Nutrition Facts
Serving Size 1/2 cup (55g)
Servings Per Container about 8

Amount Per Serving	Cereal	Cereal with 1/2 cup Skim Milk
Calories	240	280
Calories from Fat	60	60
	% Daily Value	
Total Fat 0g	0%	0%
Saturated Fat 0g	0%	0%
Cholesterol 0mg	0%	0%
Sodium 70mg	3%	6%
Total Carb. 40g	13%	15%
Dietary Fiber 3g	12%	12%
Sugars 19g		
Protein 4g		

▷ **Know Your Terms**

Labeling	Amount Per Serving
Low saturated fat	1 gram or less of saturated fat
Low fat	3 grams or less of fat
Low cholesterol	20mg or less of cholesterol and 2 grams or less of saturated fat
Low sodium	140mg or less of sodium
Low calorie	40 calories or less
Lean	Less than 10 grams of fat 4.5 grams or less of saturated fat Less than 95mg of cholesterol
Extra lean	Less than 5 grams of fat Less than 2 grams of saturated fat Less than 95mg of cholesterol

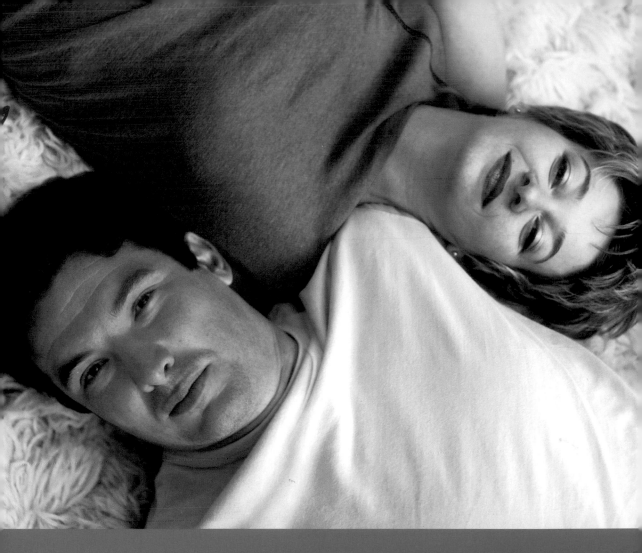

Different People,
Different Diets

**Every diet plan has something different to offer,
so choose a plan that's a "natural fit" for you.**

A Closer Look at Some
Popular Diet Plans

Every diet plan has something different to offer, so make sure to choose a plan that's a "natural fit" for you. Here are some important guidelines to help you make the right selection:

☑ First and foremost, consider your health needs.

Your personal health issues are probably the most important consideration when choosing a diet plan. Many diets (including the Healthy Living Plans at eDiets.com) have been designed to help you control a specific health condition, such as heart disease or diabetes. These plans follow the dietary guidelines established by leading health authorities such as the American Heart Association.

☑ Find the plan that's closest to your "natural" way of eating.

Your diet should include foods that you like to eat, so you can follow it without feeling deprived. If you prefer to eat smaller meals throughout the day, don't choose a diet that's based on three daily meals. If you enjoy eating carbs, find a plan that includes healthy carbs, like whole grains.

☑ Make sure the diet fits your lifestyle.

If you don't want to cook, stay away from recipe-based plans that will require you to spend more time in the kitchen. If you're a person who constantly eats on the run, go for a convenience plan that includes microwaveable foods or prepared foods.

☑ Get help if you need it.

If you feel that you need more help to make the right decision, consult a professional. Speak to your doctor or a nutrition professional. Or log on to www.eDiets.com and we'll help you find the plan that's right for you.

Glycemic Impact Diet™

GLYCEMIC IMPACT DIET™

THE BOTTOM LINE	Lose weight and body fat without feeling hungry and improve overall fitness by eating a healthy balance of 40% carbs, 30% protein and 30% fats.

The Glycemic Impact (GI) Diet has been hailed as the easiest, healthiest way to achieve long-term weight loss. The plan, which traces its roots to Canada but recently gained amazing momentum in England, is now taking America by storm.

Experts agree that of all the "celebrity diets" on the market, the GI Diet seems to have the best science behind it. In fact, some studies indicate the GI Diet can even lower your risk for heart disease and diabetes.

▷ The GI Diet Theory, in a Nutshell

The Glycemic Impact Diet is based on research that shows people who eat more high-fiber foods and fewer nutrient-dense foods lose weight more successfully. And they keep it off longer.

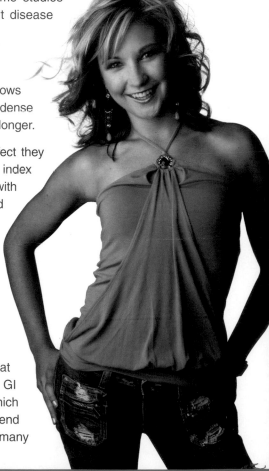

The 0-100 glycemic index ranks foods based on the effect they have on blood sugar levels. Foods with a low glycemic index value slowly release sugar into the blood, providing you with a steady supply of energy and leaving you feeling satisfied longer so that you're less likely to snack. Foods with a high GI value cause a rapid, short-lived rise in blood sugar. This leaves you tired and hungry within a short period of time. The result? You end up reaching for a snack. If this pattern is repeated often, you're likely to gain weight by constantly overeating.

▷ Feel Fuller Longer

Diets based on the glycemic index encourage you to eat foods with a low GI value and avoid those with a high GI value. This helps to prevent swings in blood sugar, which helps you feel fuller longer. Most GI diets also recommend cutting down on fat, especially saturated fats. This means many of the foods that have a low GI value but are high in fat will still be limited on the plan.

Eat lower-calorie, higher-volume foods such as vegetables, clear soup and fruit, whole grains and whole-grain cereals and breads, and you will feel satisfied. You'll eat fewer calories and lose weight without feeling hungry.

It helps your body slow digestion and absorption, so you feel fuller longer.

The Glycemic Impact Diet helps your body slow digestion and absorption, so you feel fuller longer. It also helps you sustain energy levels throughout the day, stabilize blood sugar levels and avoid carbohydrate cravings.

Highly processed, high-glycemic index foods, including white bread and pasta, sugary cereals, mashed potatoes and white rice, are replaced with vegetables and fruits, legumes, unprocessed grains including oatmeal, and long-grain brown rice. This healthy meal plan also includes low-fat and nonfat dairy, lean meats and healthy fats, including monounsaturated fat from olives and avocados, plus omega-3 fatty acids from fish, nuts and seeds.

▷ How It Works

The Glycemic Impact Diet achieves stable blood sugar and energy levels by:

— Providing approximately 40 percent of calories from unrefined, complex carbohydrates, including whole grains and whole-grain breads and cereals, and whole fruits rather than fruit juices

— Balancing carbohydrates with 30 percent of calories from lean protein (including fish, chicken, and occasionally beef and pork) with vegetarian options that include soy protein, tofu and textured vegetable protein

— Designating about 30 percent of calories for healthy fats, including nuts, fatty fish, avocados and olive oil

— Providing the same healthy mix of balanced 40-30-30 nutrition at every meal

The Glycemic Impact Diet represents the ultimate in healthy eating by excluding refined carbs, simple sugars, and saturated and trans fats. Some meals may be slightly higher in fat or protein or lower in carbohydrate, but at the end of the day, your total nutritional balance is maintained as designed with a healthy 40/30/30 mix.

The Glycemic Impact Diet stabilizes blood sugar levels throughout the day by providing your body with healthy, balanced meals and snacks every four to five hours. Your personal calorie requirements will determine whether you get two or three snacks daily.

Anxious to see what kind of food you can eat on the Glycemic Impact Diet? Check out this sample menu:

Sample Menu

Breakfast: Vegetable omelet with wheat bread & strawberries

Lunch: Grilled cheese and tomato sandwich with salad & milk

Afternoon Snack: Roast beef roll-ups with flatbread

Dinner: Chicken Florentine with brown rice & fruit

Late-Night Snack: Yogurt with raspberries & almonds

Bill Phillips'
Eating for Life™

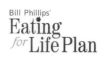

THE BOTTOM LINE	Get healthy, boost energy and lose fat by feeding your body, not starving it. Enjoy a "cheat day" once a week without compromising your program!

Have you relied on deprivation — maybe even starvation — to drop those extra pounds? Maybe you followed a strict regimen of unappealing, flavorless foods … and you lost weight. But after a while, your weight loss came to a grinding halt. Before long, you buckled under the pressure, returned to your "normal" eating habits and started packing on the pounds again.

▷ Eat Six Times a Day

Fitness superstar Bill Phillips has witnessed this dangerous diet cycle time and time again, and it's the subject of his best-selling book, *Eating for Life*. His satisfying diet and fitness routine lets you eat six times a day while you lose weight and keep it off for the long-term.

"Eating for Life really opens people's eyes to the wide variety of foods that can be enjoyed on a healthy meal plan," Phillips says. "Food is really your body's natural ally … not an enemy. The secret is learning to work with food, not against it."

According to Phillips, Eating for Life doesn't cut calories or eliminate any food groups. In fact, his way of eating isn't based on high- or low-anything. Instead, Phillips uses the three B's to describe this meal plan: basic, balanced and best. Because the body needs protein, carbohydrates and essential fats, Phillips

believes people eventually will find a happy medium that includes a healthy balance of all the macronutrients.

"Eating for Life is based on feeding the body rather than starving it," Phillips says. "I think a lot of the old diets were based on the idea of reducing food intake as a method of producing weight loss. Now, we're realizing it's the quality of your nutrition that's important. I think the key is the right portions and the right combinations."

The key to Phillips' plan is eating the right foods in the right portions and the right combinations at the right times.

"People need to look at becoming healthy and fit instead of just losing weight."

What can you eat on the Eating for Life plan? Just about anything, says Phillips. You'll enjoy beef, chicken, fish, eggs, reduced-fat dairy products, whole-grain pastas, bread and rice. You'll also eat a wide variety of vegetables, and you can indulge in many of your favorite meals, like Mexican and Italian-inspired dishes. Help yourself to traditional American foods — from chicken soup to steak and potatoes — because on Phillips' plan, these are all great choices.

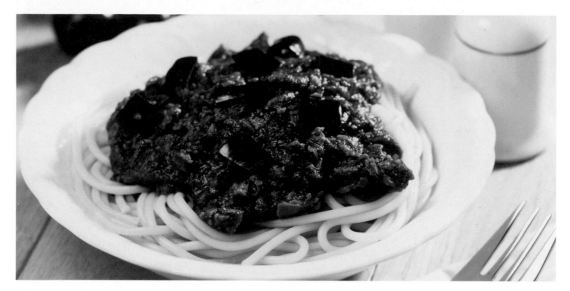

▷ Eat, Cheat, Lose!

Now here's the really unique part of this meal plan: the weekly cheat day. Once a week, you can eat anything you want as long as you return to your regular eating plan the next day. For the weary dieter, the weekly "cheat" day can provide a welcome break from the rules. Deprivation has been the undoing of many successful diets. But if you allow yourself to indulge once a week, you'll be more likely to stick with your meal plan longer.

Eating for Life is also a balanced way of eating that yields results. Follow the proven plan and you'll lose 1 to 2 pounds of body fat per week.

▷ Energize Yourself

"It's designed to help you lose fat, not just weight," Phillips says. "You'll see a steady reduction in body fat. Second, on the emotional side, you'll feel more energetic. You'll feel more like exercising. You'll feel more at peace with the issue of food instead of feeling like you're in a fight or frustrated with it."

Phillips' first program, Body for Life, was a great way to get started, as it taught people

positive habits. Now, Eating for Life builds upon that structure, establishing healthy eating as more of a lifestyle. Phillips points out that having the right mindset is key, especially when it comes to exercise.

"People need to look at becoming healthy and fit instead of just losing weight. Your aspiration should be making your body fit, strong, and energetic instead of smaller. That's where I like to see people focus. To do that, you need to provide your body with quality nutrition and feed it what it needs and then realize exercise has to come into play. Exercise can take many different forms. It has to be there at least 20 minutes, 5 days a week."

Sample Menu

Breakfast: Curried eggs with pita & fruit

Mid-meal #1: Chicken cranberry salad

Lunch: Steak on toast with side salad

Mid-meal #2: Mini corned beef sandwich with carrots

Dinner: Turkey ragout with pasta

Dessert: Very berry chocolate pudding

New
Mediterranean Diet™

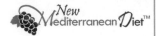

THE BOTTOM LINE	**This food-lover's diet brings back bread, pasta, fruit ... even wine! It can help you lose weight, lower cholesterol and reduce your risk for heart disease and cancer.**

It's easy to see why the traditional Mediterranean-style diet has received so much acclaim. It has been called the world's healthiest eating regimen because you can enjoy great foods — and the occasional glass of wine — while fighting disease and triggering weight loss.

▷ Proven Success

Diets may come and go, but the super-tasty Mediterranean way of eating has remained steadfast for thousands of years, according to researchers who consider it the original, the best and the only way of eating you'll ever need for a longer, healthier life.

"While some fats promote good health, others are increasingly being linked to disease," says eDiets' Chief Nutritionist Susan Burke. "The Mediterranean Diet provides optimal amounts of healthy fats to keep your immune system strong, while promoting taste and satisfaction."

The New Mediterranean Diet is a rich source of essential fatty acids and antioxidants, which can help improve cholesterol levels and protect heart health. For years, scientists have known that people who live in countries bordering the Mediterranean Sea enjoy longer, healthier lives, and they attribute much of this phenomenon to the traditional Mediterranean diet.

▷ Significant Health Benefits

In June 2003, the *New England Journal of Medicine* published research showing that people who follow the traditional Mediterranean lifestyle enjoy a lower risk for heart disease and some cancers, as well as longer life spans.

Unlike today's Western diet, which is high in unhealthy trans and saturated fats, the Mediterranean people, from Spain and Portugal on the west all the way to the Middle East, traditionally consume an unrefined plant-based diet with moderate amounts of fish and poultry, wine and occasional sweets.

Make healthy food choices without sacrificing flavor or variety.

In the Lyon Heart Study, published in the February 1999 issue of *Circulation: Journal of the American Heart Association*, research showed that heart attack victims who adopted a Mediterranean diet reduced their risk of a second heart attack by 50 to 70 percent compared to those eating a "Western-type" diet.

"In the late '80s and '90s, fat-free meal plans dominated the weight-loss industry," Burke says.

"But large, well-controlled studies show that people who eat healthy fats from fish, plant oils, nuts and seeds enjoy longer, healthier lives."

▷ What It Can Do for You

This healthy lifestyle which originated in the Southern countries bordering the Mediterranean Sea — Southern Italy and France, Greece, Spain and Portugal — can also help you lose weight. Rich in fresh, whole foods, the New Mediterranean Diet is a way of life that favors quality over quantity. Follow it correctly and you'll take the time to savor your food, and find the time for daily heart-strengthening activity. The best part is that it can help you keep your weight under control.

"Fat plays many important roles in our diet," Burke says. "Most importantly, fat tastes good. When you enjoy your diet, even if you're restricting calories, you're more satisfied."

This healthy meal plan is very much about satisfaction. It lets you make healthy food choices without sacrificing flavor or variety. A Mediterranean diet is a plant-based program that features whole, fresh foods like fruits and vegetables, nuts, fish, olive oil and satisfying whole grains. Meals and recipes are tasty and simple to prepare. Processed and refined foods, convenience foods and fast foods are avoided in a Mediterranean diet. It also eliminates trans fats and "bad" fats like butter.

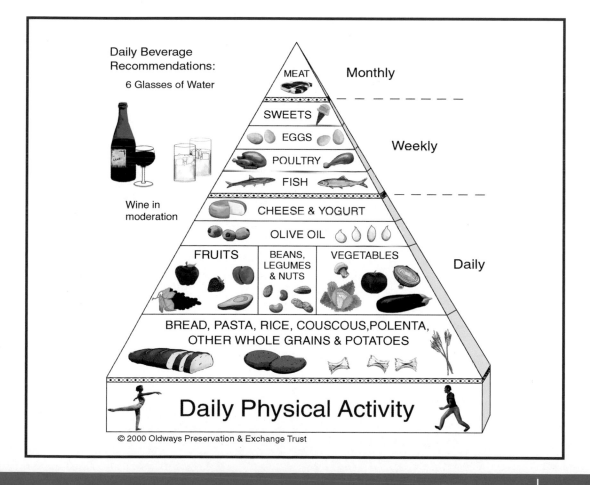

Daily Beverage Recommendations:
6 Glasses of Water

Wine in moderation

MEAT — Monthly

SWEETS
EGGS
POULTRY
FISH — Weekly

CHEESE & YOGURT
OLIVE OIL

FRUITS | BEANS, LEGUMES & NUTS | VEGETABLES — Daily

BREAD, PASTA, RICE, COUSCOUS, POLENTA, OTHER WHOLE GRAINS & POTATOES

Daily Physical Activity

© 2000 Oldways Preservation & Exchange Trust

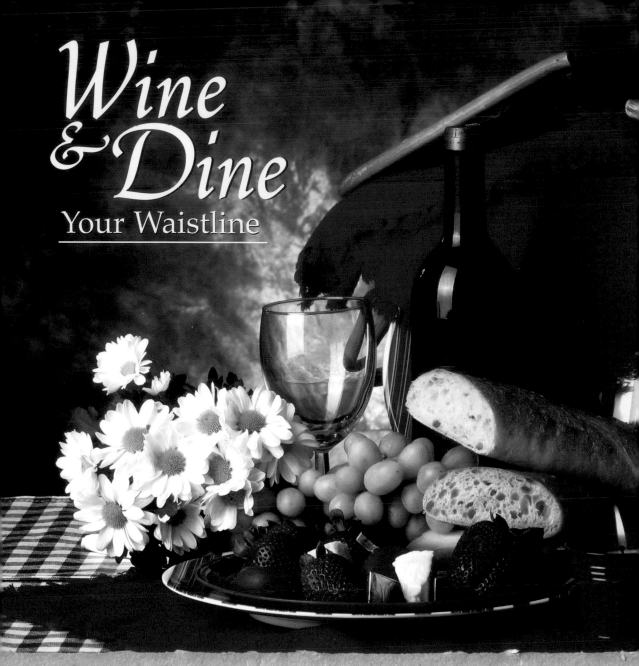

Wine & Dine

Your Waistline

People who eat a traditional Mediterranean diet enjoy a wealth of health benefits including weight loss.* A true "food-lover's diet," this plan is rich in whole grains, unprocessed foods and "good" fats. It includes delicious, satisfying foods like bread, fruit and pasta, and even wine in moderation.

The NEW Mediterranean Diet ...

do it for life!

Start by losing 10 lbs. in 5 weeks!

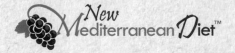

**New England Journal of Medicine*, June 2003 © 2006 eDiets.com, Inc. eDiets and eDiets.com are registered trademarks of eDiets.com, Inc. All rights reserved.

The **Mediterranean Diet Pyramid**, presented by the Oldways Preservation Trust, is based on the traditions of Crete and southern Italy in the 1960s.

The pyramid is a guide to healthy eating. It illustrates how often foods should be eaten and their importance in the diet. For example, red meat is positioned at the narrow top of the Mediterranean pyramid, to be eaten infrequently. Just below is a grouping of other animal proteins — fish, poultry and eggs — to be eaten weekly (or a few times weekly in the case of fish).

Here's what you can eat:

▷ Daily

— Eat plenty of vegetables and fruit; also include potatoes, whole-grain breads, cereals, pasta and rice; dried beans, legumes, nuts and seeds.

— Eat low to moderate amounts of cheese and yogurt (low-fat and nonfat versions are preferable).

— Eat fresh fruit as dessert.

— Replace butter, margarine and other vegetable oils with olive oil as your primary fat.

▷ Weekly

— Eat fish several times weekly and skinless poultry less often. Eat up to four egg yolks per week (including those used in cooking and baking).

▷ Occasionally

— At most, red meat should be eaten only once or twice per month, not to exceed 12 to 16 ounces per month.

— Limit sweets and saturated fats to only a few times per week.

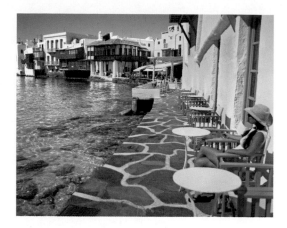

▷ Optional

— You may enjoy moderate consumption of wine on this diet, normally with meals. Men may have two 5-ounce glasses daily; women may have one 5-ounce glass daily. (Wine is not recommended for anyone with a medical condition where alcohol is contraindicated, or for those who don't currently drink alcohol.)

The Mediterranean lifestyle also encourages regular physical activity to help you:

- Maintain optimal weight
- Increase strength and fitness
- Reduce stress
- Promote endurance

Sample Menu

Breakfast: Cheddar cheese toast with milk & dried fruits

Lunch: Argentinian stuffed chicken with balsamic green beans, brown rice & an orange

Snack: Strawberry-pineapple shake

Dinner: Grilled salmon with baked potato, lemon broccoli & kiwi

The **Blood Type** Diet®

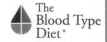

THE BOTTOM LINE	This plan offers four individual diets based on your biological profile and blood type.

Chicken, tomatoes, kidney beans, wheat – these foods sound like the foundation of a healthy diet. But some of the foods you think might help your weight-loss efforts may actually hinder your progress. That's the philosophy behind the Blood Type Diet, the meal plan based on the best-selling book *Eat Right 4 Your Type* by doctor of naturopathy, Peter D'Adamo, ND.

While plenty of weight-loss programs can be tailored to your wants and needs, how many are designed with your blood type in mind?

D'Adamo says his Blood Type Diet provides a personalized plan based on your unique blood type (A, B, AB or O). In fact, he calls his innovative, ground-breaking approach to weight loss the first post-modern diet.

▷ **Blood Type and Food**

According to D'Adamo, certain foods contain lectins (proteins), which interact with your body in different ways according to your blood type. When you eat foods containing lectins that are incompatible with your blood type, the lectins interfere with digestion, metabolism and your immune system, making you sick, tired and fat.

D'Adamo simplifies the science by grouping foods into three main categories (beneficial, neutral and avoid) for each individual blood type. Take a close look at some of the foods that fall into the "avoid" category, and you'll be surprised to see many "healthy" foods.

For example, people with Type O blood should avoid cauliflower, leeks, yucca, potatoes and cucumber. Lectins interact in different ways according to blood type.

Essentially, that means if you don't have a working knowledge about which foods impact your blood type, you may think you're eating healthfully when you really aren't. And it's not just your weight that pays the price. By tailoring your eating habits to your blood type you have the ability to improve your overall health, says D'Adamo.

Foods are grouped into 3 main categories: Beneficial, Neutral & Avoid.

"You have control with this plan," he says. You can get phenomenally good results by having

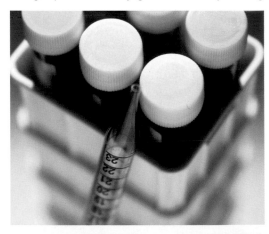

the knowledge of what's right and what's wrong for you. And you don't have to follow the diet 100 percent to get dramatic results.

If you want to control illness and maximize weight loss, keep your compliance level high. Ninety percent of your foods should come from neutral or beneficial foods. This will move a person very far, very fast.

Unlike other diet plans that are based on a specific prototype, like low-fat or low-carb, this diet is predicated on the exact relationship between your blood type and a particular food. It identifies fats that are bad for a specific blood type. It's the natural evolution of the way diets are going. If you're Type B, turkey is acceptable, but chicken is an "avoid" because of the lectin in the organ and muscle meat. While most people would lump the two birds into the same flock of foods, there's a big difference in how they affect different blood types.

Are you eating right for your blood type?

▷ Type O

Foods that encourage weight gain: Wheat, corn, gluten, kidney beans, navy beans, lentils, cabbage, Brussels sprouts and cauliflower

Foods that encourage weight loss: Kelp, seafood, iodized salt, liver, red meat, kale, spinach and broccoli

Tips for Type O: Emphasize animal proteins; focus on anger management; engage in aerobic exercise to reduce stress

▷ Type A

Foods that encourage weight gain: Meat, dairy foods, kidney beans, lima beans and wheat

Foods that encourage weight loss: Vegetable oils, soy foods, vegetables and pineapple

Tips for Type A: Vegetables are important; practice stress management (yoga or gentle exercise); take naps or frequent breaks to help you stay focused

▷ Type B

Foods that encourage weight gain: Corn, lentils, peanuts, sesame seeds, buckwheat and wheat

Foods that encourage weight loss: Green vegetables, meat, liver, eggs (low-fat) dairy products and licorice tea

Tips for Type B: Vary your diet; focus on creative outlets; engage in walking and meditation to reduce stress

▷ Type AB

Foods that encourage weight gain: Red meat, kidney beans, lima beans, seeds, corn, buckwheat and wheat

Foods that encourage weight loss: Pineapple, tofu, seafood, dairy, green vegetables and kelp

Tips for Type AB: Eat smaller, more frequent meals; focus on cultivating your natural spiritual tendencies; break up your day with physical activity to feel more energized

Sample Menu

Breakfast: Tofu apple-pear scramble

Lunch: Dill tuna salad on greens with pineapple juice

Snack 1: Pineapple spritzer & walnuts

Dinner: Curried leg of lamb with mango ginger chutney & basmati rice

Snack 2: Creamy peach drink

Atkins
Nutritional Approach™

THE BOTTOM LINE	The original low-carb plan can help stabilize your blood sugar, lower cholesterol and address many other obesity-related medical conditions.

Unless you've been marooned on a deserted island for the past 30 years, you probably know of someone who has tried — and has succeeded with — the Atkins approach to dieting.

Dr. Atkins first became a key player in the field of weight loss when he released his best-selling book *Diet Revolution* in 1972. Despite a hailstorm of criticism, the plan has not only survived, it has thrived in the past 30 years.

Weight loss without deprivation is definitely compelling, and many proponents of this proven nutritional approach attribute their success to satisfying foods on the Atkins plan. According to Colette Heimowitz, Nutritional Director of Education and Research at Atkins Health and Medical Information Services, you can say goodbye to that fat forever ... IF you follow the diet the way it's supposed to be done.

▷ The Four Phases of Atkins

The Atkins plan proclaims the key to lasting weight loss is keeping track of carbs, not calories. White flour and white sugar are off-limits because Atkins believes they could be a major cause of America's out-of-control obesity epidemic.

The first phase of the Atkins Nutritional Program sets the stage for you to reach your weight-loss goals. Induction is designed to jump-start your weight loss, end your carbohydrate cravings and stabilize blood sugar levels. Phase I lasts a minimum of 14 days and will switch your body chemistry to burning primarily fat for energy rather than carbohydrate. The Induction Phase is most restrictive as far as carbs are concerned. However, as you move into the other phases of Atkins, you add preferred carbs (some fruits, vegetables, seeds and nuts) back into your diet.

▷ Satisfying Foods

Studies show that Atkins dieters can expect to lose six to 20 pounds in their first two weeks. And they do so while eating the very foods that most weight-loss plans eliminate (like meat and butter).

When you eat more carbs, you crave more carbs. It becomes a vicious cycle.

"What's beautiful about the Atkins approach is that you can eat luxuriously," Heimowitz says. "You can have lobster with butter, steak and Caesar salad without the croutons. You can go into a diner and have bacon, eggs and sausage."

Heimowitz says many people have the

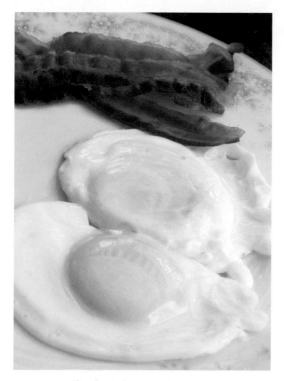

mistaken belief that the Atkins plan calls for massive meat consumption. But fresh fish, poultry, vegetables, fruits, cheeses and whole grains are also featured, so the Atkins approach can be easily adapted to your lifestyle and food preferences.

▷ Bye-Bye Cravings

"You don't have to count calories on this plan. You only have to count carbohydrates," Heimowitz says. "People who follow the Atkins Nutritional Approach find they're not as obsessed with food, and their appetites are much more controlled. When they follow Atkins, they lose those annoying cravings for sweets and carbohydrates. Their energy is much improved because they avoid the roller coaster ride of high/low blood sugars, which occurs when excessive carbs are consumed. Their body composition changes, too. Their clothes fit them better. They lose inches. That's

because the majority of weight lost is fat mass."

Heimowitz is quick to point out that not all carbohydrates are created equal. If you follow the Atkins plan, that doesn't mean you'll spend the rest of your life avoiding carbs. You'll simply need to eliminate the unhealthy carbs and replace them with healthy ones.

"The Atkins Nutritional Approach works for people who need to control carbohydrate consumption so their body can burn fat," Heimowitz says. "It's for people who suffer from carbohydrate addiction, for people who are overweight and for those who are not as physically active as they need to be. Atkins is for anyone who's looking for permanent weight control."

Though the Atkins Nutritional Approach may not be for everyone, Heimowitz says it is ideal for many groups of people, including those who carry most of their weight around their middle, those who feel sleepy shortly after eating, dieters who are always hungry and obsessed with food, people who have hypertension and high triglycerides, and those who are insulin-resistant.

What can you eat on Atkins? See for yourself with this sample menu:

Sample Menu

Breakfast: Fried eggs, bacon, Atkins bread & butter

Lunch: Roasted chicken, baked brie with sun-dried tomato & salad

Snack: Open-faced roast beef sandwich with mayonnaise

Dinner: Southwestern pork chop with green beans

eDiets.com®
Weight-Loss Plan

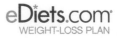

| THE BOTTOM LINE | This diet is flexible enough to fit your life and personalized to your natural way of eating – so it's easier to follow. |

Everyone is different. There is no one diet that works for everyone. That's why this personalized meal plan is built specifically for you and your needs. Whether your goal is more energy or reaching optimal health, the eDiets Weight-Loss Plan will help you reach your goal and maintain it. You determine the kinds of food you want to eat and the lifestyle choices that will work for you.

▷ What Can I Eat?

The weekly menus deliver balanced nutrition based on your individual tastes. For example, if you prefer not to eat red meat, fish or eggs, they will be excluded from your weekly menus.

▷ A Perfect Fit

Next, you'll choose the lifestyle option that best fits your life. The eDiets Weight-Loss Plan gives you three different lifestyle options.

If you're time-challenged or don't like to cook, the convenience plan has easy-to-prepare, healthy foods from your local supermarket, and healthy options for eating on the run, including fast food.

If you like to cook, try the recipe plan with quick meals that can be scaled easily to feed a family. Recipes are included for all your meals, plus a convenient "print-and-go" shopping list.

If you need different things from your meal plan at different times of the day, the combination plan is for you. It provides you with the flexibility to eat convenience foods for breakfast and lunch while you prepare delicious meals for dinner.

Regardless of which option you choose, it will have the correct caloric parameters for your needs. Whether you like to cook, hate to cook or just can't find the time, the eDiets Weight-Loss Plan will give you exactly what you need — even a fast-food option.

▷ Do It for Life

Once you've hit your goal weight, you'll be asked whether or not it is the weight at which you want to stay, or if you want to continue to lose more weight within your healthy weight range. If you decide to stay at the weight you have reached, then you will begin a healthy maintenance plan.

Sample Menu

Breakfast: Hot cereal with walnuts, honey, fruit & milk

Lunch: Healthy squash & tempeh casserole with salad & fruit

Snack: Low-fat muffin & herbal tea

Dinner: Grilled marinated steak with broccoli-cheese potato

Find your perfect diet.

No two people are exactly alike. That's why **the same diet won't work for everyone.** You need a personalized diet that suits your lifestyle and your tastes. Because a diet that "fits" you is easier to <u>live</u> with … and <u>lose</u> with.

The Diet Needs Analysis™
This amazing new diet-matching technology can help you find the diet that's right for you. And here's the best part … it's absolutely FREE.

Find the diet that fits your life … not someone else's!
Log on to www.eDiets.com and find your perfect diet.

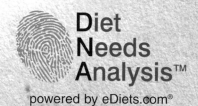

Diet
Needs
Analysis™

powered by eDiets.com®

© 2006 eDiets.com, Inc. eDiets, eDiets.com, and Diet Needs Analysis are registered trademarks
or trademarks of eDiets.com, Inc. ® or ™ as indicated. All rights reserved.

Healthy Living Plans
from eDiets.com®

Weight management and healthy living go hand in hand. So if a diet doesn't address your specific health concerns, then it may not be the best fit for your lifestyle.

Your main health concern right now may simply be to lose weight. But to accomplish that weight loss, you need a program that will address any additional health problems you have. High blood pressure, high cholesterol or food allergies are conditions that will help determine which diet plan is right for you. Be sure to consult with a physician to make sure you select a plan that can satisfy your dietary needs.

eDiets.com offers 10 different **Healthy Living Plans** designed to help you control a specific health condition or meet a special food preference, like vegetarian or dairy-free. These plans emphasize prevention and make it easier for you to plan and prepare healthy meals by providing weekly menus with shopping lists.

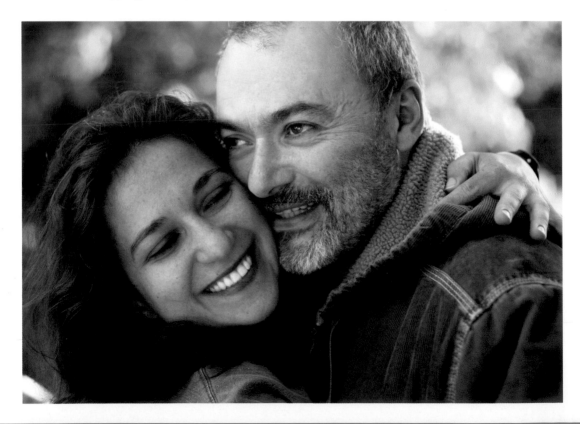

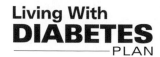

Living With DIABETES PLAN

THE BOTTOM LINE | This nutritionally balanced, carb-controlled plan helps control blood sugar levels & improve health.

Scientific advances have made great inroads into controlling this serious disease. Proper nutrition and a healthy meal plan will help you control diabetes. Work with your healthcare provider and follow a proper nutrition plan, and you can live a longer, healthier, happier life.

50% Carbohydrates
25-35% Protein
25-35% Healthy Fats

Type 2 diabetes is the most common form of diabetes, and obesity is a major risk factor. With Type 2 diabetes, either the body does not produce enough insulin, or the cells ignore the insulin. Proper diet is essential to reduce your risk for complications like amputation. Not only can a proper diet help you shed unwanted pounds, it will also keep your blood sugar levels under control, reduce your risk for heart disease, maintain your energy levels and control your cravings for sweets.

▷ Balance Is Key

A good plan will contain the same amount of carbohydrate at every meal and snack to help stabilize blood sugars. A diet based on the American Diabetes Association guidelines is best. Each meal should contain 50 percent carbohydrates, 25 to 35 percent protein and 25 to 35 percent healthy fats.

Your diet will include a variety of foods, especially those containing a high amount of fiber, like whole-grain breads and cereals, vegetables, beans and fruits.

▷ The Truth About Sugar

A common misconception is that people with diabetes should never eat sugar. However, the American Diabetes Association changed its nutrition guidelines in 1994 to allow people with diabetes to consume foods containing sugar in moderation.

Eating healthful food, exercising regularly and monitoring your blood sugar level will help you avoid the problems that make the consequences of diabetes so serious.

▷ Stay Active

Regular exercise is essential. People with diabetes should check their blood sugar before and after exercising and consult their physician before beginning a new fitness program.

If you want to follow a weight-loss program, it is essential that you review your plan and your medications with your doctor before you begin. As you continue to lose weight and your body changes, your needs will change as well. So continue to stay in close touch with your healthcare provider.

Sample Menu

Breakfast: Apple banana shake & almonds

Lunch: Traditional tuna sandwich, salad & fruit

Snack: English muffin melt

Dinner: Steak & broccoli stir-fry with brown rice & fruit

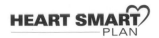
THE BOTTOM LINE	This plan follows the American Heart Association's guidelines to reduce unhealthy fats & lower your risk of heart disease.

Do you have a family history of heart disease? Are you overweight? If so, you should follow a heart-healthy diet program. A good plan includes foods that are low in cholesterol, saturated fat and sodium. It should be flexible with satisfying foods that won't leave you feeling hungry.

▷ The Number One Killer

Heart disease is the leading cause of death in America. The American Heart Association says one in three women will die of heart disease or stroke. In fact, women are more likely to die from heart disease than from cancer, chronic lung disease, pneumonia, diabetes, accidents and AIDS combined.

▷ What You Can Do

You have the power to defeat heart disease. The most important changes you can make are: quitting smoking, decreasing high cholesterol, reducing high blood pressure, becoming physically active and maintaining a healthy weight.

It is also essential to give your body the right balance of foods. If you suffer from elevated cholesterol levels, high blood pressure or have a family history of heart disease, it is important to follow a diet based on the American Heart Association's daily recommendations with no more than 30 percent of total calories from fat — of which less than 10 percent comes from saturated fat. It should have less than 300 milligrams of dietary cholesterol, less than 2,400 milligrams of sodium, and it should be high in fiber.

This diet will help you reduce your intake of foods that are high in saturated fat and dietary cholesterol with low-fat alternatives, such as lean meats and low-fat dairy products. You will eat more foods that help lower LDL ("bad") cholesterol, such as whole grains, vegetables, fruit, beans, oats and cereals, all of which are low in saturated fat and contain no cholesterol. You'll also eat heart-healthy monounsaturated and polyunsaturated fats, including olive oil, avocados and nuts, and Omega-3 fatty acids from fish.

Quit smoking, lower your cholesterol & blood pressure, get active and control weight.

In fact, the higher your blood cholesterol level, the greater your risk for developing heart disease or having a heart attack. Angioplasty and Coronary Artery Bypass Graft (heart bypass surgery) are generally the result of clogged arteries and blocked blood flow.

High blood cholesterol itself does not cause symptoms, so you may not know that your cholesterol level is too high. Lowering cholesterol levels can help reduce your risk of heart disease.

Sample Menu

Breakfast: Raspberry-banana protein shake with peanut butter & crackers

Lunch: Grilled chicken sandwich with healthy fries, salad & fruit

Snack: Popcorn medley

Dinner: Vegetarian tofu & mushroom pasta Italiano with salad & fruit

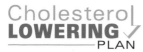
Cholesterol LOWERING ✓ PLAN

THE BOTTOM LINE | This healthy eating plan lowers bad cholesterol by eliminating unhealthy fats from your diet.

Fast food and other highly processed meals aren't good for us. A Cholesterol Lowering Plan will focus on heart-healthy, tasty foods, such as Mediterranean salmon salad and whole-grain cereals and breads. The plan can reduce the risk for heart disease and lower cholesterol, and it cuts bad dietary fats. While dairy causes problems for some, fast food and other highly processed meals aren't good for any of us.

Sample Menu

Breakfast: Whole-grain cereal with nonfat milk & fruit

Lunch: Mediterranean salmon salad with bread, fruit & yogurt

Dinner: Turkey burger on bun with healthy fries, fruit & salad

Snack: Popcorn & juice

LOW-FAT PLAN

THE BOTTOM LINE | This heart-healthy plan cuts dietary fat to help you lose weight, lower cholesterol & improve digestion.

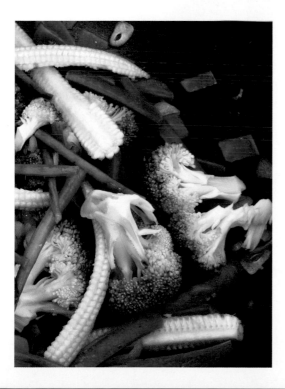

Another cholesterol reducer, the Low-Fat Plan also enhances heart health. It can also bring relief to those who suffer from indigestion, acid reflux and gallstones. Use this plan to lose weight sensibly and improve your overall health. Low-fat doesn't have to be low on flavor – enjoy beef stir-fry, plenty of fruit and savory snacks on this plan, not to mention lots of other great foods.

Sample Menu

Breakfast: Soy yogurt with nugget cereal, wheat germ, almonds & fruit

Lunch: Beef & tomato kabobs with baked potato, salad & fruit

Dinner: Shrimp fried rice with fruit

Snack: Pita chips with tofu salsa

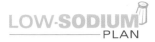

LOW-SODIUM PLAN

If high blood pressure is a concern, you should cut back on salt and sodium. Following a Low-Sodium Plan can help reduce your chances of heart disease and stroke by improving heart function and reducing fluid retention.

This plan replaces salt with vinegar, spices and herbs, such as oregano, garlic and onion. Try chicken with spinach sauce or Melba toast with soy nut butter.

Sample Menu

Breakfast: Oatmeal with rice milk, almonds & raisins

Lunch: Caribbean-style baked fillet of fish, rice, salad & fruit

Dinner: Grilled marinated steak with baked sweet potato, salad & fruit

Snack: Half a peanut butter sandwich

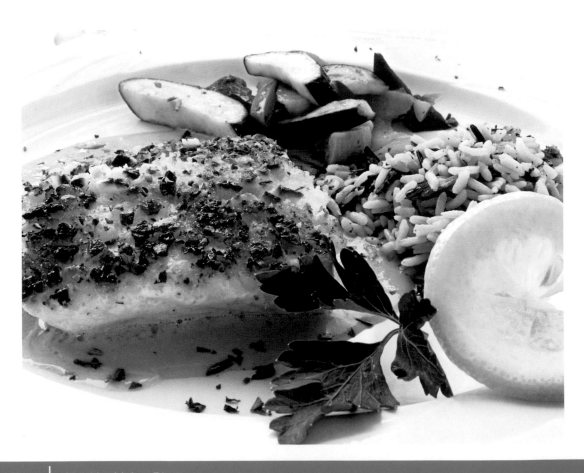

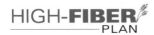

The High-Fiber Plan lowers cholesterol, improves bowel function and digestion, and reduces risk for colon cancer. Research has shown that a diet high in fiber can reduce your chances of getting certain types of cancer and help you feel satisfied longer. The plan offers recipes that include whole grains, beef and pepper sauté with rice pilaf, as well as crunchy tuna salad and low-fat cheese.

Although some red meat is high in saturated fat and cholesterol, which can raise your blood cholesterol, you do not need to stop eating it or any other single food. Red meat is an important source of protein, iron and other vitamins and minerals. You should, however, cut back on the amount of saturated fat and cholesterol you eat. One way to do this is by choosing lean cuts of meat with the fat trimmed. Another way is to watch your portion sizes and eat no more than 6 ounces of meat a day. Six ounces is about the size of two decks of playing cards.

Sample Menu

Breakfast: Hot cereal with walnuts, honey, cinnamon, rice milk & fruit

Lunch: Teriyaki pita pocket & fruit

Dinner: Pork & pepper saute with rice pilaf

Snack: Half a sliced chicken breast sandwich

HEALTHY SOY PLAN

Whether you are vegetarian or at risk for heart disease, the Healthy Soy Plan may be a good match for you. It helps you eat less animal-based protein, reduces risk of heart disease and increases healthy antioxidants. The health benefits of soy are indisputable, but if you think you have to eat bland tofu to get more in your diet, think again. This plan calls on a variety of foods, like Cuban-style rice and beans and Asian tofu burgers.

Sample Menu

Breakfast: Spiced hot cereal with walnuts, fruit & milk substitute

Lunch: Spicy beef kabobs with brown rice, salad & fruit

Dinner: Hamburger on a bun with fruit & salad

Snack: Popcorn medley

Challenge: Frequent dining out	Start Weight: 158 lbs. End Weight: 118 lbs. Pounds Lost: 40

Results not typical.

The GI Diet Helped Kim Drop 40 lbs.

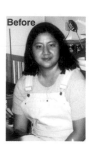

Before

For curvy-again Kim M., 40-30-30 proved to be her lucky numbers. After college, the 32-year-old media buyer's affinity for dining out and her aversion to healthy, home-cooked meals became a growing problem. Eventually the number on the scale peaked at 158 pounds. It was a heavy burden for Kim to drag around on her petite 5'2" frame — mentally and physically.

She tried her luck at a popular weight-loss center, but it wasn't a good fit for her. After seven weeks on the program, her total loss amounted to a measly four pounds.

It wasn't long after finishing a meal that she would become tired and hungry again. The vicious cycle never seemed to end. Kim constantly felt like she was running on empty. But that all changed when Kim followed the GI Diet.

For Kim, the GI Diet was the solution she'd been searching for. After so many failed attempts, Kim could've called it quits. Instead, she put her faith in a more novel approach that met her nutritional needs.

Looking back, Kim says following the GI Diet was the best thing she ever did for her health.

"I had read that a plan like this would increase my energy and provide me a more balanced way of eating. I couldn't believe how easily I lose the weight and how I've managed to keep it off."

Although she still dines out a couple of times a week, the GI Diet got her in the habit of making her own meals. One secret to success was shopping around the perimeter of the supermarket. She mainly buys meats and vegetables instead of processed foods.

After a couple of weeks following the healthy eating plan, Kim says she could feel the change in her body and the boost in her energy levels. In addition to altering her diet, she added regular exercise to her daily routine. Her regimen included Spinning twice a week, two to three days of weightlifting, running and some yoga.

The one-two punch of healthy eating and regular fitness accomplished what exercise alone couldn't do. The dramatic results kept her plugging along throughout the process.

"I feel good about my body," Kim notes. "I'm more energetic. People have been amazed by my results. Now, when I look at the old pictures, I can't believe that was me. It never will be again."

WE'LL DO
THE COOKING ...

YOU'LL LOSE
THE WEIGHT!

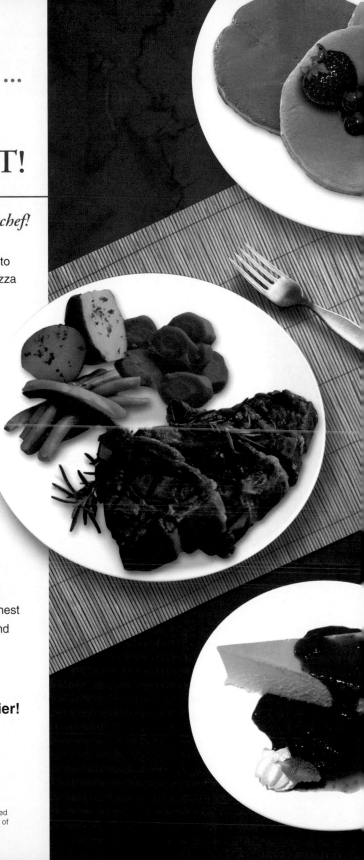

It's like having your own personal chef!

It's not always easy to eat right. If you hate to cook, or life's just too busy, fast food and pizza delivery could be the downfall of your diet.

Easy does it

Now you can enjoy *fresh* gourmet meals, *delivered* directly to your door with the eDiets Fresh Cuisine plan. Select from a menu of nutritionist-approved meals that fit your diet plan.

Imagine ... No planning. No measuring. No shopping. No cooking. And no clean-up. Just *heat* and *enjoy*. It doesn't get any easier than that.

Taste the difference

Not only is our Fresh Cuisine delivery plan simple ... it's simply delicious! Your *fresh* meals are *chef-prepared* using only the finest quality ingredients and no preservatives. And our unique packaging process keeps your weekly meals fresh in your refrigerator.

Meal delivery makes dieting easier!

FRESHCUISINE™

Healthy Meals Delivered by eDiets.com®

© 2006 eDiets.com, Inc. eDiets and eDiets.com are registered trademarks of eDiets.com, Inc. Fresh Cuisine is a trademark of eDiets.com, Inc. All rights reserved.

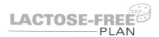
LACTOSE-FREE
——— PLAN

A Lactose-Free Plan helps those who suffer from lactose intolerance, which is the inability to digest significant amounts of lactose, the predominant sugar in milk.

This inability results from a shortage of the enzyme lactase, which is normally produced by the cells that line the small intestine. Milk and other dairy products are a major source of calcium nutrients in the American diet. The Lactose-Free Plan replaces milk and dairy products with other calcium-rich foods for balanced nutrition.

Sample Menu

Breakfast: Roast beef toast with soy milk & fruit

Lunch: Chicken sandwich with salad & fruit

Dinner: Southwestern spicy frittata, with salad & fruit

Snack: English muffin with soy butter

Hypoglycemia/
LOW-SUGAR
——— PLAN

THE BOTTOM LINE | This plan helps stabilize blood sugar levels, control sugar cravings & reduce mood swings.

A Hypoglycemic/Low-Sugar Plan helps stabilize blood sugar, control cravings for sweets and reduce mood swings. People suffering from hypoglycemia worry about experiencing sugar crashes and the physical effects they cause.

This plan is designed to eliminate those tired feelings, and it is delicious. On a given day, you can eat cereal with milk and walnuts, along with toast and jelly for breakfast. Later you might have chicken rolls in mushroom sauce, rice pilaf and salad. Grilled, marinated steak with broccoli-cheese potatoes may be the menu for dinner, with whole-wheat pretzels and club soda for a snack. And fruit accompanies nearly every meal. This plan is set up so that dieters get enough carbohydrates, which are the main dietary source of glucose.

Sample Menu

Breakfast: Cereal with milk & cottage cheese with blueberries & walnuts

Lunch: Moroccan chicken salad with couscous & fruit

Dinner: Peanut butter sandwich, creamy fruit shake & salad

Snack: Cheesy pita chips with club soda

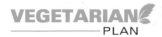
Many people who become vegetarians do so for health reasons. But what can following a vegetarian meal plan do for you? Since a vegetarian diet tends to be low in saturated fat, high in fiber and rich in vitamins and minerals, vegetarians generally have a lower risk of heart disease and some cancers.

▷ The Meat of the Matter

By cutting higher-fat meats from your meals, you'll eliminate some of the saturated fat that can lead to clogged arteries and raise your risk for heart disease. It will also eliminate extra calories, which can help with weight loss. And because you're eating more vegetables and fruits, you're likely to take in more phytochemicals and fiber, which can help lower your risk for heart disease and certain types of cancer.

Vegetarians don't have to eat soy products if they don't want to. There are plenty of other veggie protein sources besides soy, including eggs and low-fat dairy products.

If you like meat but want to eat mostly vegetarian, you needn't worry. In fact, if you choose the right cuts and try to limit your consumption to only a few times per month, meat provides high-quality protein and iron. Red meats that are lean, such as sirloin, typically make a good lower-fat beef choice.

Finding suitable substitutes for your favorite meat products might just take some creativity. Almost every meat and dairy product has an alternative, from hot dogs and sausage to meatballs, yogurt and pudding. Most of these products contain protein because they're made with soy. And many are lower in fat than the original versions, so check the label.

▷ How Strict Are You?

Vegetarians differ widely in their strictness. Which of the following labels best describes the type of diet you plan to follow?

Semi-vegetarian: Eats dairy, eggs, poultry and fish, but no other animal products.

Pesco-vegetarian: Eats dairy, eggs and fish, but no other animal products.

Lacto-ovo vegetarian: Eats both dairy products and eggs, but no other animal products.

Lacto-vegetarian: Eats dairy products, but no eggs or other animal products.

Vegan: Eats no meat, poultry, fish, eggs or other animal products.

Sample Menu

Breakfast: Vegetarian bacon with toast, yogurt & fruit

Lunch: Linguine Florentine with fruit & salad

Dinner: Tofu & bean enchiladas with fruit & salad

Snack: Cottage cheese with fruit cocktail

Diet Checklist

Now that you've read up on some of the more popular diets, here's a handy checklist for you to compare them.

	Fat Controlled	Carb Controlled	Exercise Program Available
eDiets.com WEIGHT LOSS PLAN	✔		✔
Jenny Craig®	✔		
NEW! GLYCEMIC IMPACT DIET™	✔ (emphasis on healthy fats)	✔	✔
Weight Watchers®			
New Mediterranean Diet™	✔ (emphasis on healthy fats)		✔
NutriSystem®		✔ (available)	
South Beach Diet™	✔ (bans unhealthy fats)	✔	
Bill Phillips Eating for Life™	✔		✔
L.A. Weight Loss Centers®		✔ (depends on plan phase)	
The Blood Type Diet®	✔ (depends on blood type)	✔ (depends on blood type)	✔
TRIM KIDS™	✔		✔

Color indicates plan available at eDiets.com.

Kid Friendly	Support Available	Dining Out OK	Flexible Meal Plan	Meetings Available	Special Food Required
	✔	✔	✔	✔	
	✔			✔ (counseling)	✔
	✔	✔	✔	✔	
	✔	✔	✔	✔	
	✔	✔	✔	✔	
	✔				✔
	✔	✔	✔		
	✔	✔	✔ (free cheat day)	✔	
		✔			(supplements suggested)
	✔		✔	✔	
✔	✔	✔	✔	✔	

The information in this chart is based on the latest public information available at press time and may not reflect any recent changes to the plan. For more information about a specific plan, please contact that company directly. eDiets and eDiets.com are registered trademarks of eDiets.com, Inc. Jenny Craig is the registered trademark of Jenny Craig, Inc. Weight Watchers is the registered trademark of Weight Watchers International, Inc. Nutrisystem is the registered trademark of Nutri/System IPHC, Inc. The South Beach Diet is the registered trademark of SBD Trademark Limited Partnership SBD Trademark, Inc. L.A. Weight Loss Centers is the registered trademark of L.A. Weight Loss Centers, Inc.

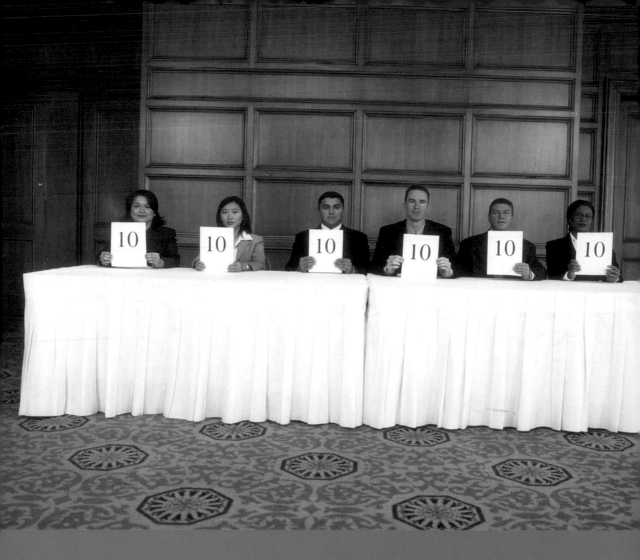

Simply the **Best**

These Top 10 Lists can help you make those healthy everyday choices that mean so much.

Eat to Lose: 10 Best Fat-Burning Foods

Best Fat-Burning Foods

1	Water
2	Green tea extract
3	Soup
4	Grapefruit
5	Apples & pears
6	Broccoli
7	Low-fat yogurt
8	Lean turkey
9	Oatmeal
10	Hot peppers

Stoke your metabolic fire and burn calories faster with these diet-friendly foods and beverages. Just remember: Calories count, portion control rules, and there's no substitute for a well-balanced diet and regular exercise.

Water accelerates weight loss. A German study showed subjects increased their metabolic rates (the rate at which calories are burned) by 30 percent after drinking water. It is also a natural appetite suppressant that banishes bloat as it flushes out sodium and toxins.

Studies show **green tea extract** boosts metabolism and may aid in weight loss. This mood-enhancing tea also contains anti-cancer properties and helps prevent heart disease. It's also a trendy favorite among weight-conscious celebrities.

Eat less and burn fat faster by having a bowl of **soup** as an appetizer or a snack. A Penn State University study proves soup is a super appetite suppressant. Women in the study who ate soup consumed 100 fewer calories than those who chose a chicken and rice casserole (or the casserole and a glass of water).

The **grapefruit** diet is not a myth. Researchers at Scripps Clinic found that participants who ate half a grapefruit with each meal in a 12-week period lost an average of 3.6 pounds. The study indicates that the unique chemical properties in this vitamin C-packed citrus fruit reduce insulin levels and promote weight loss. *NOTE: If you are taking medication, check with your doctor about any potentially adverse interactions with grapefruit.*

Overweight women who ate the equivalent of three small **apples or pears** a day lost more weight on a low-calorie diet than women who didn't add fruit to their diet, according to researchers from the State University of Rio de Janeiro. Fruit eaters also ate fewer calories overall. Eating fruit helps you feel full longer and eat less.

Study after study links calcium and weight loss. **Broccoli** is high in calcium and loaded with vitamin C, which boosts calcium absorption. It also has plenty of vitamin A, folate and fiber. And, at just 20 calories per cup, this weight-loss superfood not only fights fat, but also contains powerful phytochemicals that boost your immunity and protect against disease.

Dairy products can boost weight loss efforts, according to a study in *Obesity Research*. People on a reduced-calorie diet who included 3-4 servings of dairy foods lost significantly more weight than those who ate a low-dairy diet with the same number of calories. Low-fat yogurt is a rich source of calcium, providing about 450 mg (about half the recommended daily allowance for women ages 19-50) per 8-ounce serving and 12 grams of protein.

Rev up your fat-burning engine with a bodybuilder favorite, lean **turkey**. Protein can help boost metabolism, lose fat and build lean muscle tissue so you burn more calories. A 3-ounce serving of boneless, skinless, lean turkey breast weighs in at 120 calories and provides 26 grams of appetite-curbing protein, 1 gram of fat and 0 grams of saturated fat.

Oatmeal is a heart-healthy favorite that ranks high on the good carb list because it's a good source of cholesterol-fighting, fat-soluble fiber (7 grams per 3/4-cup serving), which keeps you full and gives you the energy you need to make the most of your workouts. Choose steel-cut or rolled oats, not instant oatmeal, to get your full dose of vitamins, minerals and fiber.

Eating **hot peppers** can speed up your metabolism and cool your cravings, researchers at Laval University in Canada found. Here's why: Capsaicin (a chemical found in jalapeño and cayenne peppers) temporarily stimulates your body to release more stress hormones, which speeds up your metabolism and causes you to burn more calories.

Here's how these 10 fat-blasting superstars help you lose weight:

- Each of these healthy weight-loss boosters fills you up and keeps you full longer on fewer calories.

- Water-rich fresh fruits, veggies and soup dilute the calories in your food and allow you to eat more without breaking the calorie bank.

- High-fiber fruit, vegetables and nutritious whole grains keep your digestive system on track and steady your insulin levels, which prevents fat storage.

- Lean meat boosts metabolism and burns calories because it takes more energy to digest than other foods.

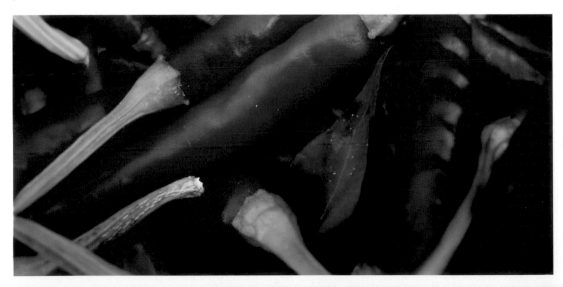

10 Healthiest Foods **for Kids**

Healthiest Foods for Kids

1	Oatmeal
2	Eggs
3	Nut butters
4	Yogurt
5	Melon
6	Broccoli
7	Sweet potatoes
8	Protein
9	Whole grains
10	Orange juice

Childhood obesity rates are soaring, and parents need to take action. Kids can be finicky, so parents need to work harder to make healthy eating a habit. These 10 foods can help.

WARNING: Allergies can prevent a normally healthy food from being a healthy food for any child. This is a general list to help you choose healthy foods for your children without allergies. If you have questions about food allergies, seek advice from your healthcare provider.

Oatmeal is full of B vitamins, iron, zinc and calcium. It offers quick energy for busy kids with its carb load and fiber count.

Eggs are a great source of protein and nutrients, including B vitamins, vitamin E and zinc. The American Heart Association's guidelines have changed to include an egg a day for adults. There are no formal recommendations for children, other than limiting their cholesterol intake to 300mg per day. An egg is equivalent to 213mg, so use your best judgment.

Nut butters are great fast foods for kids. While peanuts can be problematic or life-threatening for children with allergies, other nut butters may be OK (but check with your pediatrician first).

Yogurt is a great source of calcium, and it's easier to digest than regular milk. The cultures (check the label to make sure they're in there) are beneficial to good colon health, especially if your child has been on antibiotics. Watch the sugar content, though.

Melon is rich in vitamin C, beta-carotene and bits of B vitamins. Trace minerals and calcium fill every juicy bite. Melons are not to be missed when they're plentiful and in season.

Kids like to call **broccoli** "trees," and sometimes you can get picky kids to eat trees rather than broccoli. Broccoli is one of the best vegetables for adults and growing kids, providing calcium, potassium, beta-carotene and B vitamins.

Sweet potatoes contain 30mg of beta-carotene per cup. (It would take 23 cups of broccoli to get that same amount!) They provide three grams of fiber per serving.

Kids need **protein** to keep growing. Good choices include legumes, beans (combined with a grain to make a complete protein), soy products like tofu, or lean meat, fish or poultry.

The best nutrition is found in **whole grains**. Brown rice and whole-wheat bread are a quantum leap over their white counterparts and offer necessary fiber, minerals and vitamins.

Orange juice is full of vitamin C, vitamin E, potassium, folate and zinc.

Top 10 Foods **for Women**

Best Foods for Women

1	**Beans**
2	**Kale**
3	**Beta-carotene**
4	**Flaxseed**
5	**Iron**
6	**Soybeans**
7	**Water**
8	**Broccoli**
9	**Calcium**
10	**Salmon**

Striking a nutritional balance in our stressed-out lives has never been more important — especially for busy women. To stay in control, women need to eat right. Start with these 10 super foods:

Beans are nutritious, low in fat and easy on the budget. Beans pack more than 5 grams of fiber in only one half-cup serving – that's a whopping 25 percent of your daily allowance.

Kale is loaded with folate, an important B vitamin for women (you need 400 micrograms daily). A folic-acid deficiency during pregnancy may cause neural-tube defects in babies.

Beta-carotene, a precursor to vitamin A, is found in orange squashes, pumpkin, butternut squash and sweet potatoes. This important nutrient may help reduce the risk of breast cancer and helps repair your skin.

Flaxseed and flaxseed oil are full of omega-3 fatty acids, which may help protect women from heart disease and painful arthritis. The fiber in flax comes from lignans, which are now being studied for their role in cancer prevention.

Women should get more **iron** from food sources. The type of iron found in food is much easier for the body to absorb than iron in pill form. Lean red meats, dark poultry and lentils are some of the best sources of iron.

Phytoestrogen-rich **soybeans** can help women significantly lower bad cholesterol (LDL) and raise good cholesterol (HDL). Tofu is a great source of soy protein.

Water is a nutrient, and we need plenty of it. Water suppresses the appetite and helps the body metabolize stored fat.

Broccoli is a fabulous source of calcium and contains other important nutrients like potassium and a good smattering of B vitamins. It's also one of the best foods for children, so enjoy it as a family.

Women need to increase their **calcium** intake. The Recommended Daily Allowance is 800mg a day, but some experts say that most women should get 1,200 to 1,500mg a day. When you take into consideration the epidemic of osteoporosis among older women, it might not be a bad idea to increase your dairy intake. A good choice is yogurt.

Weight-conscious women used to choose white fish or sole over salmon. Now that we understand the value of omega-3 essential fats, it's time to get serious about salmon. **Salmon** is high in protein, low in cholesterol and contains quite a few B vitamins, calcium, zinc, iron and magnesium.

10 Best **Canned Foods**

Best Canned Foods	
1	Tuna
2	Beans
3	Tomatoes
4	Chili
5	Spaghetti sauce
6	Vegetable soup
7	Salsa
8	Applesauce
9	Evaporated milk
10	Fruits & veggies

When you're short on time and trying to get dinner on the table, there are few things quicker than canned foods. While many canned foods are high in sodium, there are quite a few good choices on your grocer's shelves. Just read the nutrition labels. Most canned foods can stay on your shelf for up to two years.

Try these top 10 favorites:

Naturally low in fat and high in protein, water-packed tuna is a healthy favorite. (Because tuna can be high in mercury, some health experts advise pregnant or lactating women to avoid it.) Choose solid albacore, which offers great taste.

Beans are low in fat, and high in fiber and nutrients. Canned beans offer convenience without soaking. The Goya brand carries a wide variety that makes it easy to mix it up.

Canned tomatoes offer extra phytochemical power in the form of lycopene, a proven antioxidant that may lower the risk of certain diseases, including cancer and heart disease. The redder the tomato product, the stronger the benefits.

Many canned chilis are a quick, easy, satisfying meal — the hard part is choosing just one. Look for chilis that contain lots of beans, lean meat and low sodium.

There are few things quicker than canned foods.

Spaghetti sauce is hardly worth making from scratch anymore. Taste-test a few canned versions, and you'll save time without sacrificing flavor.

Low-sodium vegetable soups are a terrific way to keep hunger at bay with a satisfying combination of tasty broth and fiber-filled veggies.

Canned and jarred salsas have come a long way. Some are so incredible that your friends won't believe you didn't spend hours chopping and mixing. And don't forget those beneficial phytochemicals that tomatoes pack!

Applesauce is delicious by itself and is a great substitute for oil or butter in baking. Remember to choose an applesauce that has no sugar added.

Evaporated milk is made for cooking and baking, but some people use it as a rich coffee creamer. Try the non-fat varieties.

Buy canned fruits and veggies in low-sodium or no-sodium varieties. Be sure to choose fruits that are packed in water, not syrup.

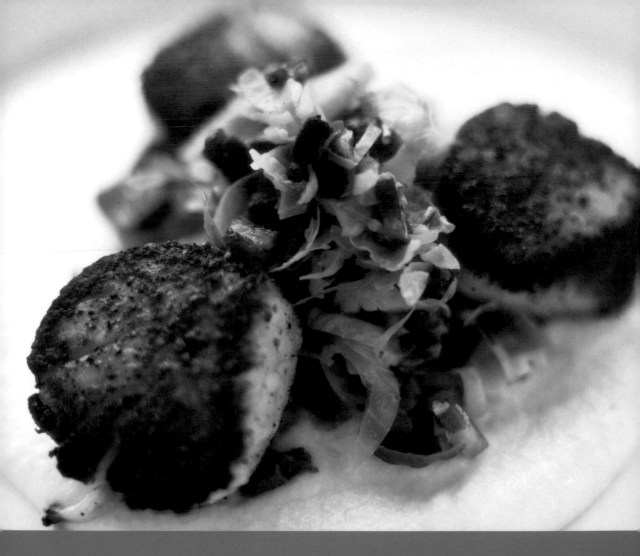

Scrumptious Meals,
Simple Recipes

What's cooking in your kitchen? Try some of
these easy-to-make healthy favorites!

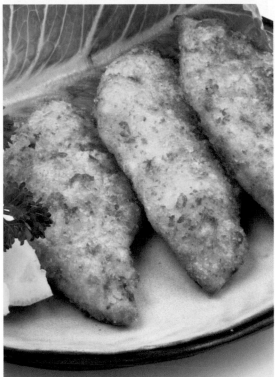

Crispy Baked Fish

Ingredients

4 fresh fillets of fish of choice (5 1/2 oz. each)
1/2 cup milk substitute
1/2 cup dairy-free, low-fat or nonfat Parmesan cheese
3/4 cup low-sodium breadcrumbs
1 tsp. paprika
1 cup liquid egg whites

Directions

Preheat oven to 450 degrees. Rinse and pat dry fish. Set aside. In a medium bowl, combine liquid egg whites and milk substitute. In a separate bowl, combine Parmesan cheese, breadcrumbs and paprika. Dip fish into egg mixture, then dredge fish into breadcrumb mixture; coat fish evenly. Arrange fish on a baking sheet or shallow pan. Discard any extra egg and breadcrumb mixture. Bake about 5 minutes or until fish flakes easily with a fork. Serve.

Nutritional values per serving: 333 calories, 46 grams protein, 21 grams carbohydrates, 5 grams fat (2 grams saturated fat), 621 milligrams sodium, 0 grams fiber, 3 grams sugar and 80 milligrams cholesterol.

Serves 4

Diet: **eDiets Weight-Loss Plan**

Beef Kabobs

Ingredients

4 small onions
4 bell peppers
4 garlic cloves
4 Tbsp. olive oil
1 cup white wine or white vinegar
4 tsp. thyme
1 1/4 lbs. beef, loin cut – 5 oz. portions

Directions

Rinse and trim beef of all visible fat; cut into 1-inch cubes. Cut onion into wedges, cut pepper into 1-inch squares and mince garlic. In a deep dish, combine oil, wine or white vinegar, garlic, and thyme; add beef, pepper and onion to dish. Toss to coat, cover with plastic wrap and refrigerate for at least 30 minutes. Alternately thread beef cubes, pepper and onion onto skewer. Grill or broil; turn after 4 to 6 minutes and continue grilling for another 5 to 8 minutes or until done.

Nutritional values per serving: 356 calories, 32 grams protein, 17 grams carbohydrates, 9 grams fat (3 grams saturated fat), 94 milligrams sodium, 5 grams fiber, 12 grams sugar and 75 grams cholesterol.

Serves 4

Diets: **eDiets Weight-Loss Plan, Atkins**

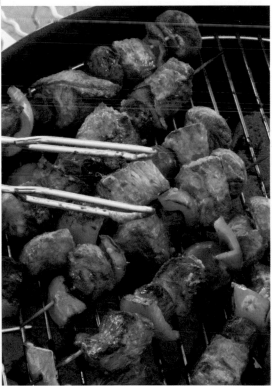

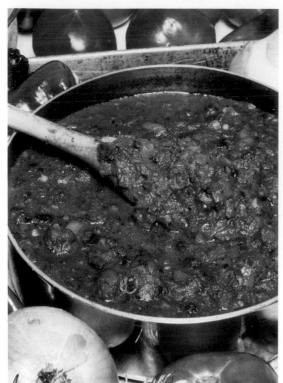

Spicy Chili con Carne

Ingredients

12 oz. lean, ground round beef
1 cup chopped onion
1 cup chopped bell pepper
2 jalapeño peppers
1 tsp. cumin
3 cups canned kidney beans, rinsed and drained
3 cups vegetable broth
2 cups low-sodium salsa
4 Tbsp. fresh cilantro

Directions

Dice jalapeño and chop cilantro; set aside. In a medium-sized pot over medium heat, cook ground beef, chopped onion, both peppers and cumin, stirring occasionally, until beef is no longer pink, about 8 to 10 minutes. Add beans, broth and salsa; reduce heat to a simmer and cook for about 10 to 15 minutes. Serve topped with chopped cilantro.

Nutritional values per serving: 257 calories, 25 grams protein, 30 grams carbohydrate, 4 grams fat (2 grams saturated fat), 740 milligrams sodium, 9 grams fiber, 7 grams sugar and 45 milligrams cholesterol.

Serves 4

Diet: **Eating for Life**

Curried Turkey Salad with Walnuts

Ingredients

1¼ lbs. boneless, skinless turkey breast
4 tsp. curry powder
1⅓ cups low-fat or nonfat, plain or sugar-free yogurt
4 cups red or green grapes
12 cups mixed salad greens
4 Tbsp. olive oil and vinegar dressing
½ cup chopped walnuts

Directions

Cut turkey into bite-sized cubes. Heat a nonstick skillet to medium high and coat with cooking spray; sauté turkey cubes 4 to 5 minutes until thoroughly cooked; remove and let cool. Mix yogurt with curry powder. Cut grapes in half. Mix cooled turkey and grapes with seasoned yogurt. Cover and refrigerate for at least 15 minutes for flavors to blend. In the meantime, rinse, dry and shred salad greens. In a salad bowl, toss greens with dressing and place on a dinner plate. Remove turkey mixture from refrigerator; place on top of salad greens. Sprinkle salad with walnuts and serve.

Nutritional values per serving: 520 calories, 46 grams protein, 44 grams carbohydrate, 21 grams fat (3 grams saturated fat), 250 milligrams sodium, 7 grams fiber, 36 grams sugar and 95 milligrams cholesterol.

Serves 4

Diets: **Glycemic Impact Diet, Eating for Life**

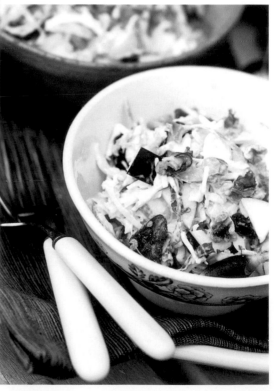

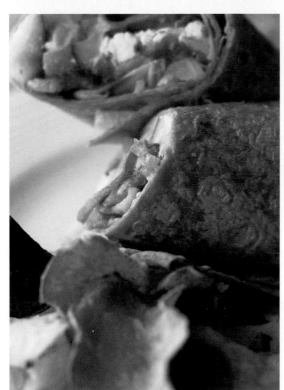

Southwestern Shrimp Wrap

Ingredients

12 oz. frozen, pre-cooked medium-sized shrimp
3 Tbsp. olive oil
2 cups frozen mixed vegetables
4 whole-wheat tortillas (approximately 6-inch diameter)
4 Tbsp. low-sodium salsa

Directions

Heat oil in a nonstick skillet on medium-high. Add veggies; stir-fry until tender but still crisp. Defrost pre-cooked shrimp according to package directions. Add shrimp to skillet with vegetables and heat through. Remove from heat. Place tortilla on a plate; spread shrimp mixture over half the tortilla and top with salsa; fold over the edge with the filling and roll it up.

Nutritional values per serving: 213 calories, 22 grams protein, 23 grams carbohydrate, 6 grams fat (1 gram saturated fat), 557 milligrams sodium, 2 grams fiber, 1 gram sugar and 167 milligrams cholesterol.

Serves 4

Diets: **Eating for Life, eDiets Weight-Loss Plan**

London Broil

Ingredients

24 oz. steak
4 Tbsp. olive oil
8 oz. red wine
4 Tbsp. fresh parsley
1 tsp. oregano
2 garlic cloves

Directions

Preheat broiler or grill. Mince garlic. In a small mixing bowl, mix together garlic, oil, wine, fresh parsley and oregano. Rinse and pat dry steak; place in a deep bowl and add marinade. Turn steak to coat all sides with marinade; cover and refrigerate at least 30 minutes, preferably overnight. Discard marinade; broil or grill meat about 4 to 5 minutes on each side or until cooked to desired doneness. Serve.

Nutritional values per serving: 363 calories, 32 grams protein, 2 grams carbohydrate, 20 grams fat (4 grams saturated fat), 93 milligrams sodium, 0 grams fiber, 0 grams sugar and 91 milligrams cholesterol.

Serves 4

Diets: **Eating for Life, Glycemic Impact Diet, Atkins Nutritional Approach**

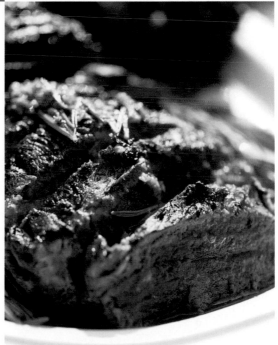

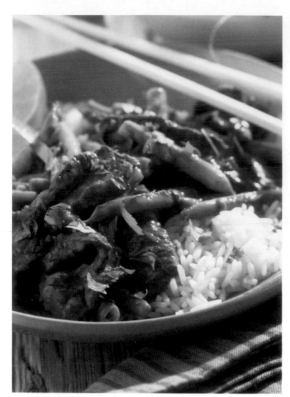

Beef Stir-Fry with Snow Peas

Ingredients

1¼ lbs. (20 oz.) beef, loin cut	4 cups chopped bok choy
4 cups fresh snow peas	4 green onions
3⅓ Tbsp. canola oil	2½ Tbsp. light soy sauce
2 garlic cloves	¼ cup sesame seeds

Directions

Slice beef into half-inch strips. Rinse all vegetables. Chop green onion, mince garlic, trim snow peas and chop bok choy into strips; set aside. In a nonstick skillet, heat oil on medium-low heat and sauté garlic for 1 to 2 minutes, until lightly golden. Raise heat to medium-high; add beef and stir-fry for 2 to 4 minutes; add all vegetables with soy sauce and stir-fry another 4 to 5 minutes until vegetables are crisp-tender. Sprinkle with sesame seeds and serve.

Nutritional values per serving: 382 calories, 35 grams protein, 10 grams carbohydrate, 22 grams fat (4 grams saturated fat), 396 milligrams sodium, 3 grams fiber, 3 grams sugar and 86 milligrams cholesterol.

Serves 4

Diets: **Eating for Life, Glycemic Impact Diet, Atkins Nutritional Approach**

Oven Chicken Nuggets

Ingredients

4 boneless chicken breasts, about 4 oz. each	2 tsp. Dijon mustard
½ tsp. paprika	¼ cup nonfat mayonnaise
½ tsp. garlic powder	1 cup breadcrumbs
1 cup enriched all-purpose flour	Cooking spray
1 cup liquid egg substitute	

Directions

Preheat oven to 375 degrees. Rinse chicken, pat dry and cut each breast into four strips. Set aside. Combine spices and flour in a large plastic zip-lock bag. Shake well. In a bowl, whisk together eggs with mustard and mayonnaise. Place breadcrumbs on a large plate.

Add chicken to the bag with flour mixture, then dip in egg mixture and roll in breadcrumbs. Place on baking pan coated with cooking spray. Bake 30 minutes until chicken is cooked through and coating starts to brown. Serve.

Nutritional values per serving: 210 calories, 31 grams protein, 14 grams carbohydrate, 2 grams fat (0 grams saturated fat), 260 milligrams sodium, 1 gram fiber, 1 gram sugar and 65 milligrams cholesterol.

Serves 4

Diet: **Trim Kids**

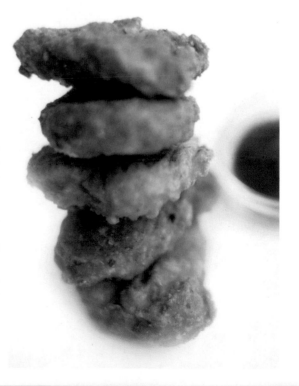

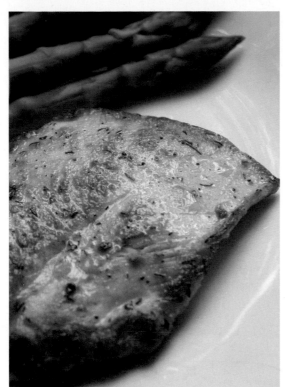

Herbed Grilled Chicken

Ingredients

4 boneless chicken breasts, 5 oz. each
1 1/3 Tbsp. olive oil
1 tsp. oregano
1 tsp. thyme
2 tsp. dried rosemary

Directions

Preheat either grill or broiler. Rinse and pat dry the chicken. Combine olive oil and herbs to form a paste and rub on chicken to coat. If possible, cover with plastic wrap and let marinate, refrigerated, for about 30 minutes. Grill or broil chicken, approximately 6 to 8 inches from heat source, for 4 to 6 minutes on each side until cooked. Serve.

Nutritional values per serving: 240 calories, 33 grams protein, 1 gram carbohydrate, 11 grams fat (2 grams saturated fat), 95 milligrams sodium, 0 grams fiber, 9 grams sugar and 80 milligrams cholesterol.

Serves 4

Diets: **Blood Type Diet, eDiets Weight-Loss Plan, Atkins Nutritional Approach**

Tropical Pineapple Slush

Ingredients

1 cup soy milk
2 scoops soy protein power
8 packets of Splenda® sweetener
2 cups pineapple chunks
1 tsp. coconut extract
4 Tbsp. sliced almonds

Directions

Drain pineapple chunks and place in a sealable freezer storage bag or plasticware; freeze overnight or longer. Before making, slightly thaw fruit for about 10 minutes at room temperature. Meanwhile, pour soy milk into blender and add protein powder and Splenda. Blend at high speed for about 15 to 20 seconds. Add pineapple and coconut extract; blend on high speed until smooth, stopping blender to scrape sides. Spoon mixture into a dessert bowl and top with almonds. Serve immediately.

Nutritional values per serving: 183 calories, 16 grams protein, 20 grams carbohydrate, 4 grams fat (0 grams saturated fat) 162 milligrams sodium, 2 grams fiber, 15 grams sugar and 0 milligrams cholesterol.

Serves 4

Diet: **Eating for Life**

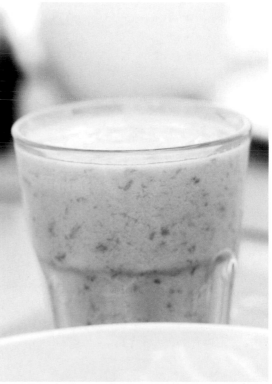

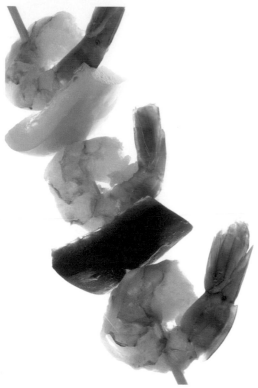

Shrimp-Vegetable Kabobs

Ingredients

1 lb. fresh or frozen
medium-sized shrimp
8 slices small onion
2 cups fresh mushrooms
20 cherry tomatoes

1 1/3 cups olive oil
6 Tbsp. fresh lemon juice
1 tsp. garlic powder
1 tsp. Italian seasoning

Directions

Preheat broiler or grill. If using fresh shrimp, peel, devein, rinse and pat dry. If using frozen, do not defrost. Peel and cut onions into wedges and set aside. Clean mushrooms with a damp paper towel. Combine oil, lemon juice, garlic powder and Italian seasoning in a bowl. Marinate shrimp and vegetables in lemon mixture, refrigerated, for at least 30 minutes. Discard marinade and alternately thread shrimp and vegetables onto skewers. Grill or broil on highest oven rack about 3-4 minutes per side until shrimp turns pink and vegetables are crisp-tender. Remove from skewers and serve.

Nutritional values per serving: 248 calories, 26 grams protein, 21 grams carbohydrate, 7 grams fat (1 gram saturated fat), 179 milligrams sodium, 3 grams fiber, 9 grams sugar.

Serves 4

Diet: **eDiets Weight-Loss Plan**

Garlic Scallops

Ingredients

24 oz. scallops
2 2/3 Tbsp. olive oil
2 garlic cloves
2 Tbsp. fresh parsley

Directions

Rinse and pat dry scallops. Mince garlic. Heat oil in a nonstick skillet to medium high heat and sauté garlic for about 1 minute. Add scallops; cook until lightly golden for 2 to 3 minutes. Be sure not to overcook. Serve sprinkled with fresh parsley.

Nutritional values per 6-ounce serving: 233 calories, 28 grams protein, 5 grams carbohydrate, 10 grams fat (1 gram saturated fat), 275 milligrams sodium, 0 grams fiber, 0 grams sugar and 56 milligrams cholesterol.

Serves 4

Diets: **Atkins Nutritional Approach,
New Mediterranean Diet**

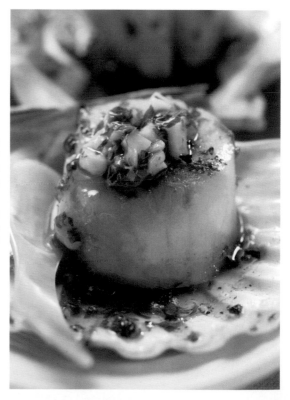

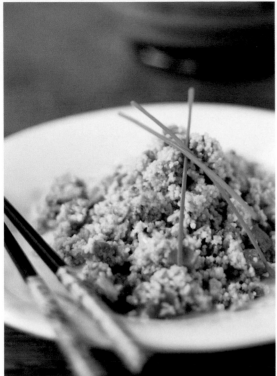

Salmon Couscous Salad

Ingredients

2 cups water	20 cherry tomatoes
1/2 cup dry couscous	4 Tbsp. olive oil
12 oz. salmon fillets, 3 oz. each	4 Tbsp. fresh lemon juice
2 cups fresh broccoli	2 garlic cloves
4 green onions	1 tsp. oregano

Directions

Bring water to a boil over high heat; remove from heat, add couscous, stir and cover. Let stand for 5 minutes. Fluff with fork and set aside to cool. Rinse and pat dry salmon. Coat a nonstick skillet with half of the oil, heat to medium high and pan fry salmon 3-4 minutes per side until no longer translucent; remove and set aside. Rinse and chop broccoli and green onion; cut the tomatoes in half. Cook broccoli in microwave or steam 3-4 minutes until crisp-tender; remove and let cool. Mince garlic and mix with remaining olive oil, lemon juice and oregano to make dressing. Coarsely flake salmon and mix with couscous and chopped vegetables. Add dressing and mix thoroughly. Serve.

Nutritional values per serving: 390 calories, 21 grams protein, 24 grams carbohydrate, 23 grams fat (4 grams saturated fat), 72 milligrams sodium, 3 grams fiber, 3 grams sugar and 50 milligrams cholesterol.

Serves 4

Diet: **Blood Type Diet**

Grilled Beef with Portabello Sauce

Ingredients

1 lb. beef tenderloin
3 Tbsp. olive oil
4 garlic cloves
4 fresh shallots
4 portabello mushrooms
1 cup vegetable broth
4 Tbsp. sherry wine

Directions

Preheat grill or broiler. Rinse and pat dry beef. Use half of the olive oil to coat beef on all sides. Grill or broil meat 4 to 5 minutes per side until cooked to desired doneness. Mince garlic and finely dice shallot; clean, trim and slice mushrooms. While beef is cooking, heat remainder of olive oil in nonstick skillet to medium high. Sauté garlic and shallot for about 2 minutes; add mushrooms and cook about 3 more minutes. Stir in broth and sherry and cook 5 to 6 minutes until liquid is reduced by half. Season to taste and serve over meat.

Nutritional values per serving: 280 calories, 25 grams protein, 8 grams carbohydrate, 13 grams fat (3 grams saturated fat), 180 milligrams sodium, 1 gram fiber, 3 grams sugar and 60 milligrams cholesterol.

Serves 4

Diet: **Atkins Nutritional Approach**

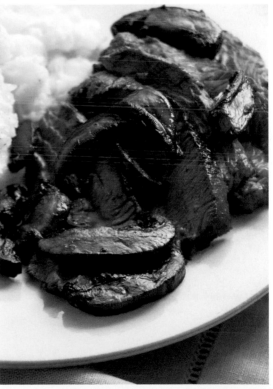

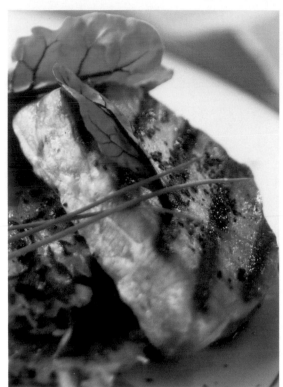

Seared Tuna with Pico de Gallo

Ingredients

4 tuna steaks (4 oz. each)	2 jalapeño peppers
4 Italian plum tomatoes	4 Tbsp. fresh cilantro
4 green onions	3 Tbsp. olive oil
2¹/2 Tbsp. fresh lime juice	1 tsp. black pepper

Directions

Rinse and dice tomato and jalapeño pepper; slice green onion and chop cilantro. In a small bowl, combine vegetables with cilantro and lime juice to make Pico de Gallo. Cover and refrigerate for flavors to blend. Rinse and pat dry tuna; rub with olive oil and season with black pepper.

Heat a nonstick skillet to high, add oil and sear tuna for about 2 minutes on one side; turn and reduce heat to medium; cook for about 5 to 7 more minutes covered for rare or medium doneness. Serve topped with Pico de Gallo.

Nutritional values per serving: 222 calories, 27 grams protein, 4 grams carbohydrate, 10 grams fat (2 grams saturated fat), 50 milligrams sodium, 1 gram fiber, 1 gram sugar and 43 milligrams cholesterol.

Serves 4

Diet: **Eating for Life**

Mediterranean Seafood Pasta

Ingredients

2 Tbsp. olive oil	8 oz. fresh or frozen
4 garlic cloves	medium-sized shrimp
2 cups fresh yellow squash	4 Tbsp. fresh basil
2 cups chopped bell pepper	4 oz. pasta, whole wheat
4 medium fresh tomatoes	4 Tbsp. fresh parsley
2 cups chopped onion	2 Tbsp. fresh, grated
8 oz. scallops	Parmesan cheese

Directions

Cook pasta per package directions, omitting any salt; drain and reserve about ¹/4 to ¹/3 cup of the pasta water; set aside. Mince garlic; rinse all vegetables and herbs. Chop squash, tomato, parsley and basil; set aside. Heat oil in a large nonstick saucepan over medium heat; sauté onion and garlic 2 to 3 minutes. If using fresh shrimp, peel, de-vein, rinse and pat dry. Defrost, rinse and pat dry if using frozen shrimp. Rinse and pat dry the scallops. Add shrimp, scallops, squash and bell pepper to saucepan; cook about 4 to 5 minutes or until shrimp is pink and scallops are opaque. Add cooked pasta with reserve liquid, chopped tomato, basil and parsley; stir to combine and heat thoroughly. Sprinkle with Parmesan cheese and serve.

Nutritional values per serving: 347 calories, 29 grams protein, 37 carbohydrate, 10 grams fat (2 grams saturated fat), 254 milligrams sodium, 7 grams fiber, 8 grams sugar and 107 milligrams cholesterol.

Serves 4

Diets: **New Mediterranean Diet, Trim Kids, eDiets Weight-Loss Plan**

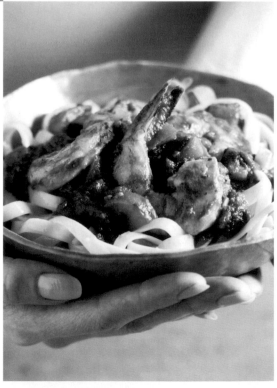

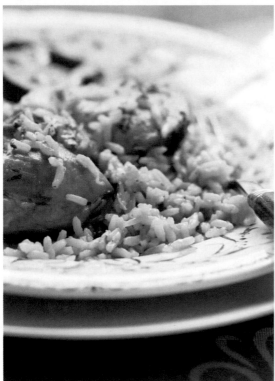

Dijon Chicken Medley

Ingredients

1 lb. boneless chicken breast (4 oz. portions)
2 1/2 Tbsp. Dijon mustard
1 cup canned kidney beans, rinsed and drained
1 cup uncooked rice
6 cups fresh spinach
5 1/3 Tbsp. olive oil
1 Tbsp. chili powder

Directions

Preheat grill or broiler. Brush chicken with mustard and grill or broil until no longer pink and cooked throughout. Cook rice according to package directions; omitting salt. Add beans, spinach, oil and chili powder to cooked rice. Stir, cover and cook at low heat until spinach is wilted, approximately 3-5 minutes. Place rice mixture on dish, add chicken and serve.

Nutritional values per serving: 554 calories, 36 grams protein, 54 grams carbohydrate, 21 grams fat (3 gram saturated fat), 369 milligrams sodium, 8 grams fiber, 1 gram sugar and 65 milligrams cholesterol.

Serves 4

Diet: **eDiets Weight-Loss Plan**

Tuna Tuscan Style

Ingredients

4 cans water-packed, low-sodium tuna (4 1/2 oz. each)
2 small onions
16 small pitted black olives
1 tsp. crushed red pepper flakes
4 cups low-sodium canned, crushed tomatoes
2 Tbsp. olive oil

Directions

Chop onion and olives; drain and flake tuna. In a nonstick saucepan, heat oil over medium heat and sauté onion until translucent, about 2 to 3 minutes. Add tuna to saucepan; add olives, canned tomatoes with liquid and pepper flakes. Partially cover saucepan, reduce heat to low and simmer for about 10-12 minutes, stirring occasionally, until most of the liquid has evaporated. Add cooked pasta to sauce, if desired (NOTE: Pasta addition will affect nutritional values); heat through, 1 to 2 minutes, and serve.

Nutritional values per serving (without pasta): 264 calories, 27 grams protein, 21 grams carbohydrate, 8 grams fat (1gram saturated fat), 243 milligrams sodium, 4 grams fiber, 8 grams sugar and 40 milligrams cholesterol.

Serves 4

Diets: **eDiets Weight-Loss Plan, New Mediterranean Diet**

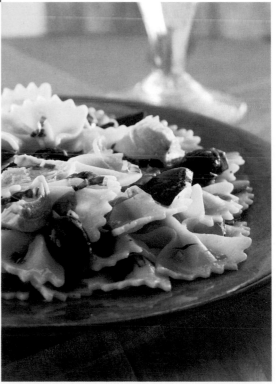

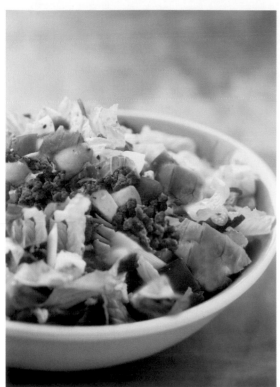

Turkey and Black Bean Salad

Ingredients

1 lb. ground, skinless turkey breast
2 tsp. taco seasoning mix
$1/2$ cup low-sodium salsa
$1 1/3$ cups canned black beans, rinsed and drained
2 medium red bell peppers
1 small red onion
4 medium fresh tomatoes
8 cups lettuce of choice, such as romaine
$1/2$ cup olive oil and vinegar dressing
2 cups peeled and chopped avocado

Directions

Heat a nonstick skillet to medium and coat with cooking spray; crumble and brown ground turkey with taco seasoning mix, stir in salsa and cook for 1 to 2 more minutes until heated through. Rinse and chop all vegetables; toss with lettuce. Add cooked ground turkey and beans to salad; top with chopped avocado and drizzle with dressing. Serve.

Nutritional values per serving: 371 calories, 35 grams protein, 36 grams carbohydrate, 13 grams fat (1 gram saturated fat), 608 milligrams sodium, 10 grams fiber, 11 grams sugar and 45 milligrams cholesterol.

Serves 4

Diets: **Glycemic Impact Diet, Eating for Life**

Tuscan Rosemary-Zucchini Omelet

Ingredients

12 large eggs
1 cup zucchini squash
4 tsp. fresh rosemary
4 oz. cheese
3 Tbsp. olive oil

Directions

Rinse and slice zucchini into thin rounds. Chop rosemary very finely. Heat oil on medium high in a nonstick skillet. When pan is hot, pour in eggs and swirl pan to cover the entire surface. Layer zucchini over one half of the skillet. Sprinkle with rosemary and cheese; cover. Cook for 3-4 minutes until set, and then using a spatula, gently fold one side over the other. Cook for 1 minute more and serve.

Nutritional values per serving: 626 calories, 43 grams protein, 7 grams carbohydrate, 45 grams fat (15 grams saturated fat), 827 milligrams sodium, 0 grams fiber, 5 grams sugar.

Serves 4

Diet: **Atkins Nutritional Approach**

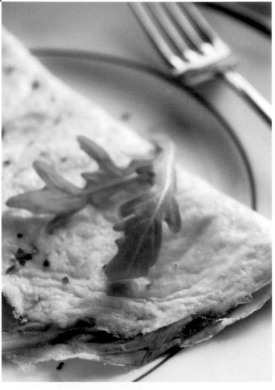

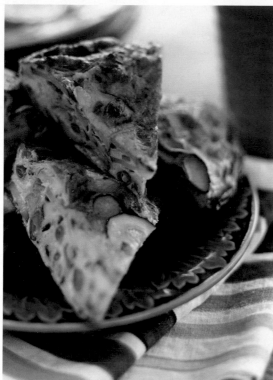

Zucchini-Tomato Frittata

Ingredients

3 cups liquid egg substitute
3 cups zucchini squash
8 Italian plum tomatoes
8 green onions
1 tsp. black pepper
1 tsp. garlic powder
2 oz. low-fat or nonfat shredded cheddar cheese
1 1/3 Tbsp. olive oil

Directions

Preheat broiler. In a small bowl, beat liquid eggs lightly with garlic powder and black pepper; set aside. Rinse and chop zucchini, tomato and green onion. Heat oil in an ovenproof skillet over medium heat and cook vegetables for about 5 to 6 minutes until zucchini is crisp-tender. Add egg mixture and cook on medium-low heat until eggs are almost set, about 5 minutes. Top with cheese and place skillet in broiler about 4 to 5 inches from the heat for about 1 to 2 minutes until cheese is melted. Serve immediately.

Nutritional values per serving: 304 calories, 30 grams protein, 19 grams carbohydrate, 12 grams fat (2.5 grams saturated fat), 440 milligrams sodium, 5 grams fiber, 11 grams sugar and 5 milligrams cholesterol.

Serves 4

Diet: **eDiets Weight-Loss Plan**

Spinach-Chickpea Salad

Ingredients

8 cups fresh spinach
1 small red onion
1 1/3 cups fresh mushrooms
2 cups low-sodium, canned chickpeas (garbanzo beans), rinsed and drained
4 Tbsp. olive oil
1/4 cup fresh lemon juice

Directions

Whisk olive oil and lemon juice for dressing and set aside. Place rinsed and dried spinach in a salad bowl. Chop onions; wipe mushrooms clean with a damp paper towel and slice. Top spinach with mushrooms, chopped red onion and chickpeas. Toss with dressing and serve.

Nutritional values per serving: 270 calories, 10 grams protein, 27 grams carbohydrate, 15 grams fat (2 grams saturated fat), 50 milligrams sodium, 7 grams fiber, 3 grams sugar and 0 milligrams cholesterol.

Serves 4

Diet: **eDiets Weight-Loss Plan**

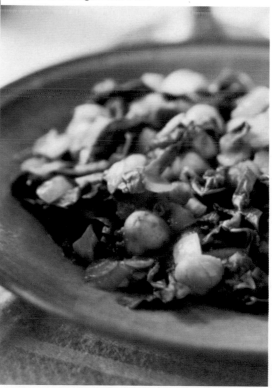

Fitness
SOLUTIONS

What's your workout style? Think about your goals, interests and resources before committing to a fitness plan.

Defining **Fitness**

A fateful time comes in everyone's life. You might be trying to get into your favorite jeans, or that special dress for a friend's wedding. That's the stomach-churning moment when you realize your clothes don't fit you anymore. So you squeeze. You wiggle. You force your body in. Then you proudly proclaim, "It still fits!"

When that moment comes, there's no denying it. You need to get in shape. But how should you do it? What makes a good fitness program?

Professional instruction can help you learn proper form and breathing and avoid injury.

Here's a definition from the President's Council on Physical Fitness and Sports: *"Fitness is the ability to perform daily tasks vigorously and alertly, with energy left over for enjoying leisure-time activities and meeting emergency demands. It is the ability to endure, bear up, withstand stress, and carry on in circumstances where an unfit person could not continue. It is a major basis for good health and well-being."*

▷ A Good Fitness Program

A good fitness program targets body, mind and spirit. It fits your current activity level and will adjust with you as you progress. If you're able, consider adding yoga, Pilates or Tai Chi to your weight-training and cardio sessions to engage your body and your mind. Include these alternative mind/body disciplines on a regular basis for complete balance. You also will want to improve cardiovascular capability, muscular strength, flexibility and

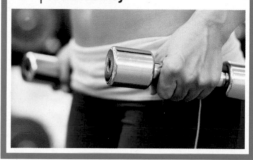

3 Basic Fitness Areas

1 | Cardiovascular Exercise
2 | Muscular Strength
3 | Flexibility

body composition for a healthier body that looks great.

Three basic areas of fitness – **cardiovascular exercise**, **muscular strength** and **flexibility** – determine your fitness level.

Typically, people do what is easiest for them or what they're good at – and that's all. This means they're ignoring the types of exercise that will ultimately do them the most good. For example, joggers might neglect strength training, and yoga devotees may not enjoy the benefits of a cardiovascular workout.

Cardiovascular exercise will strengthen the heart, lungs and respiratory system, so it is essential for good health and fat loss. During a cardiovascular workout, such as power walking or jogging, the heart, lungs and blood vessels respond by increasing the amount of oxygen available to the working muscles.

Beginners should choose an enjoyable, heart-pumping activity, such as walking or exercise tapes. You'll do best if you're consistent; start with three days per week for 20 minutes per day, and increase your workout time and frequency gradually each week.

Concerning intensity, follow the target heart rate guidelines set by The American College of Sports Medicine. These guidelines recommend that aerobic activity be performed at an intensity of 60 to 85 percent of maximum heart rate. Your target heart rate will assist with fat loss and improve energy levels.

A good fitness program targets mind, body and spirit.

To calculate your target heart rate, subtract your age from 220, then multiply that number by 0.60 to 0.85. This is a healthy range for your heart. To make tracking your heart rate easier, invest in a heart rate monitor.

For **muscular strength**, just two to three strength-training sessions with weights on alternate days of the week (no more than 30 to 60 minutes) will do the trick. Try for 8 to 12 repetitions – that's considered a good range for improving muscular strength and gaining tight, lean muscles. Do more than 12 reps, and you are primarily working toward muscular endurance.

Weight training is essential for burning body fat. For every pound of muscle you gain, your body burns 30 to 50 additional calories per day. If you gain 5 pounds of muscle, you'll be burning up to 250 additional calories per day. The cumulative effect is significant – that's more than 90,000 calories over the course of one year. Weight training also combats osteoporosis and is the shapely/sexy woman's best-kept secret.

It doesn't matter whether you use dumbbells in your home or work out at a gym; as long as the resistance is somewhat challenging, and your form is precise, you'll get good results.

Professional instruction is helpful for learning the proper form and breathing and to avoid injury.

Flexibility refers to the amount of movement that can be accomplished at a joint. A good fitness program should make stretching exercises a priority.

Tight muscles can create imbalances. Tight hamstrings (back of the leg), for example, can cause pain in the lower back and poor posture.

The following tips will improve your flexibility. Perform stretching exercises during each

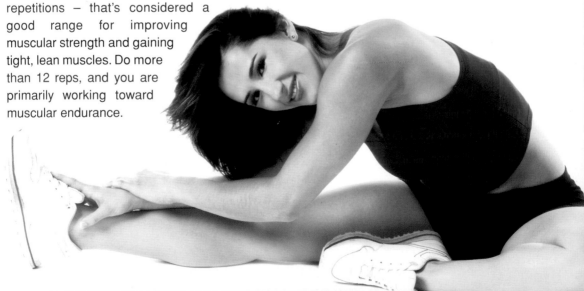

workout. Choose a few upper and lower body stretches that work all muscle groups. Stretch each area without forcing, and hold it for 5 to 30 seconds while breathing normally.

Exercise makes you feel good — and feel good about yourself.

☑ **Stretch.** Daily stretching is recommended, but if that isn't possible, you should at least stretch all of the muscles that your workout affects. Perform two to three stretches per muscle group and hold each one for 15 to 30 seconds. Always stretch to the point of mild tension, never pain. Stretching can also help alleviate chronic pain and discomfort. Surprisingly, lower back pain can be caused by tight hamstrings, which can cause an exaggeration in the curve of the back, leading to back pain. Stretch muscles often.

☑ **Use free weights.** Machines provide artificial stabilization of the core muscles. That's not to say that there isn't a place for machines in your workout. But if you use the same routine for every workout, you should mix it up with free weights, like dumbbells, so your core muscles will stabilize your body as you isolate the muscle group you're working on.

☑ **Try yoga.** Yoga not only makes you more flexible, but it also improves your balance because so much of the work requires core strength.

Body composition refers to the amount of lean tissue versus fat on your body. Lean weight is composed of muscles, bones, internal organs and other body tissue. Fat weight is just fat. A 10-minute composition test (performed at any gym) will determine the percentages. At the gym, ask for a staff member who is trained to measure body composition.

If you're eating a diet rich in protein, carbohydrates and healthy fats and following sensible strength and cardiovascular programs, chances are you're losing fat and gaining lean muscle. That means your body composition is changing. So although your scale weight may not change initially, it could be that you've gained muscle and lost fat.

▷ The Mind-Body Connection

Another reason to stick with exercise is all in your head. Many studies show that an exercise regimen can lessen depression and reduce stress, anxiety, tension and anger. Working out can assist you in working out your life's problems. Many people are convinced that exercise helps them think more clearly and that they can even find solutions to problems as they are spending time at the gym. The psychological benefits of exercise can't be overstated; it makes you feel good – and feel good about yourself.

Exercise needs to be increased in duration and intensity if results are going to continue. In that way, you not only accomplish more work and become stronger, but you also adjust your goals and set new ones for yourself.

Whatever form of exercise you choose, be sure to include fitness with your diet program for sustainable results. Be patient and follow these guidelines for a good fitness program, and you'll be well on your way to fitting into those favorite clothes again.

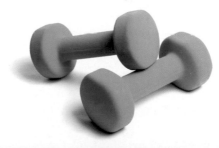

Jump-Start Your
Fitness Plan

I t's hard to make time to exercise when life gets in the way. The National Center for Health Statistics says Americans don't get enough exercise. Only 26 percent of adults engage in vigorous exercise three times per week.

Just as a good diet plan must incorporate your personal preferences and lifestyle to be successful, so must a fitness program. And while you may think that your packed schedule can't accommodate a few workouts a week, you must find a way. Exercise decreases your risk for obesity-related illnesses, such as cancer, heart disease and diabetes. It also makes you feel better and gives you energy.

Raphael Calzadilla, eDiets' Chief Fitness Pro, says "absolute" exercise recommendations don't work because they're inflexible. They view people as robots, without considering work demands, family responsibilities and personal interests. These factors must be taken into consideration. The question isn't "How much exercise?" but "How much exercise can I do each and every week to improve my health, yet stay consistent?"

▷ Start with the Basics

If you think working out involves a pricey gym membership or bulky equipment cluttering your home, think again. Your plan should include only those resources that are available to you and that you like to use. Don't worry if you're not the most coordinated or knowledgeable exerciser – just get moving and do what you enjoy.

Easy Exercise Tips

1	Push past the fear
2	Get a checkup
3	Eat healthful foods
4	Set your goals
5	Be realistic
6	Be consistent
7	Educate yourself
8	Just move
9	Beware of magic potions
10	Evaluate costs
11	Find exercises you enjoy
12	Don't get discouraged
13	Find a workout buddy
14	Enjoy music
15	Do it for life

"I've always taken great pleasure in training a beginner. Taking responsibility for your own health is a courageous and intelligent act," Calzadilla says. "Beginners learn things correctly from the start instead of re-learning the ineffective habits they picked up from an infomercial."

▷ Easy Tips to Get You Started

☑ **Push past the fear.** It's OK to feel somewhat unsure of yourself. The psychological aspect is the first thing to accept. There will be a lot to learn about weight training, cardiovascular exercise and nutrition. But as you begin the process, you'll become more comfortable and make progress.

☑ **Get a checkup.** Having a physical is a wise first step because it will help assure that you'll reap the most benefits with the least amount of risk. If you smoke, have high blood pressure, high cholesterol, diabetes or are overweight, it's doubly important.

☑ **Eat healthful foods.** Begin to get an understanding of how food affects your body. Try to understand, for example, what happens to your body when you have a big bowl of pasta. Learn how elevated blood sugar affects fat storage. Learn to monitor your portion sizes and cut calories a bit by eliminating one food each day that you know is not good for your health.

☑ **Set your goals.** Before you start exercising, decide what you want to accomplish. For example, you may decide you want to lose 30 pounds of fat and gain two pounds of muscle. Maybe you want to be able to walk five miles without losing your breath or fit into that size 8 dress. Write it down. Make it quantifiable. Just saying "I want to get in shape and lose weight" won't work because there's no defined target.

☑ **Be realistic.** Make the days when you exercise realistic for your schedule and lifestyle. Take a close look at your daily life to decide how many days and how much time you can realistically devote to exercise. This is going to be a long-term behavior pattern, so it has to be based on reality.

Many people start exercising every day thinking that's the best approach. Maybe you can only do two or three 45-minute sessions each week. It's the combination of efficient nutrition and exercise that will benefit you most, not simply excessive exercise. That's a sure way to burn out and lose interest.

☑ **Be consistent.** Maintain consistency based on your daily schedule. Get a minimum of three and a maximum of six days of exercise. One day of rest is essential. Try to exercise for a minimum of 20 minutes each session.

☑ **Educate yourself.** You'll need to develop an understanding of concepts such as repetitions, sets, cardio, etc. It is important to gain basic knowledge about these and other fitness terms.

☑ **Just move.** Start to work out. Get moving. It won't take a lot of time to do beginner's level weight training and cardiovascular exercise. During your workout, focus on form, technique, precision and breathing correctly.

☑ **Beware of magic potions.** Don't get hooked on supplements that can reduce body fat or infomercials that sell ineffective products to get your stomach flat. Remember, these companies are just trying to make a buck, and most of them don't provide all the information you require to make a wise decision.

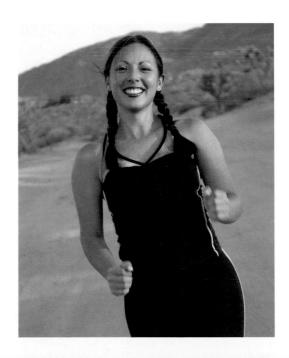

☑ **Evaluate costs.** It's important to get the most effective nutrition and workout plan for your needs. Ask yourself, "What do I get for my money?" It's also important to get ongoing education that doesn't require this to be a full-time endeavor. You need quick and timely information that won't break the bank.

Exercise decreases your risk for cancer, heart disease and diabetes.

☑ **Find exercises you enjoy.** Your exercise program can include power walking, videotapes and aerobics classes. Get creative and mix it up. If you do use videotapes and dance aerobics tapes, remember that there is no law that says you have to finish the whole tape in one session. Why not split the tape into two days (assuming it's an hour-long tape) and slightly increase your intensity level each day? You'll still get great results.

☑ **Don't get discouraged.** If you experience an exercise plateau, don't get discouraged. The truth is that everyone experiences a plateau. For some it may be two months, some six months and others longer. It doesn't matter — everyone experiences it. The point is that you need to dust yourself off and get back on your horse.

☑ **Find a workout buddy.** If you can't find a friend to work out with, post a message on your gym's bulletin board. Find someone who has similar goals and try to work out with this person at least twice per week. If you know you have to meet someone for a power walk or be at the gym or for a tennis match at a specific time, you're bound to be accountable. This tip is really valuable on those days after work when you're tempted to go home and munch on chips before dinner. Amazing things start to happen when you work out when you don't feel like working out. You increase your internal strength and dedication, and it slowly starts to catch fire.

☑ **Enjoy music.** Burn, baby, burn! CDs, that is. Make a list of the music that motivates you the most, then burn a CD with all your favorites. Studies show that people who work out to their favorite music do so longer and more intensely than those who do not. But if you're outdoors, be aware of your surroundings. Don't get caught up in the music and forget where you are.

☑ **Do it for life.** At what age will you stop working out? "Never" is a great answer. Every age group has different needs and preferences when it comes to health and wellness. You can weight train, perform cardio, stretch and compete in athletic events at any age. But as a person ages, intensity and the amount of weight lifted needs to decrease.

Are You Fit or Fat?

You are fit if you can:

- Perform daily tasks without fatigue and have ample energy to enjoy leisure pursuits
- Walk a mile or climb a few flights of stairs without becoming winded or feeling heaviness or fatigue in your legs
- Carry on a conversation during light to moderate exercise, such as brisk walking

You may be out of shape if you:

- Feel tired most of the time
- Are unable to keep up with others your age
- Avoid physical activity because you know you'll tire quickly
- Become short of breath or fatigued when walking a short distance

Source: The Mayo Clinic

Boost Your Fitness Plan
with a Healthy Diet

Food is fuel, and the human body cannot optimally respond to workouts without the healthiest foods. It's the only natural way to increase endurance, strength and lean muscle tissue. A healthy diet boosts a fitness program to new levels, while the typical fast food diet will leave your fitness program at a standstill.

For optimal performance, eat smaller, more frequent meals.

Assume two people of the same sex, height, weight, age and exercise experience are trained over the course of six months using a balanced routine of cardiovascular exercise, weight training and flexibility. One person has a healthy nutrition program. The other does not. Guess who's going to excel? The person with the nutritious diet will increase energy and strength while dramatically improving her physical appearance, compared to the poor eater.

▷ Control Blood Sugar Levels

Blood sugar control is a key factor in maintaining steady energy levels throughout the day. If you're using a program of moderate caloric intake with a balance of protein, carbohydrates and monounsaturated fats, you will experience a unique abundance of energy — probably more than you can imagine.

If your blood sugar levels consistently spike as a result of poor nutritional choices and overeating, you will most likely feel sluggish and tired, due to an over-production of the hormone insulin. One function of insulin is to take sugar out of your bloodstream and put it into your cells. When you consume excessive carbohydrates or a large meal, your blood sugar goes up. Insulin is secreted, and your blood sugar goes back down.

Do this meal after meal, day after day, and you'll feel like you have the energy of a 100-year-old person. That tired, sluggish feeling you get after a big Thanksgiving meal is a perfect example. Feed your body nutritious foods consistently, and your workout energy will increase. You'll gain strength and endurance while you reduce body fat.

If you fill up on sugar, saturated fats and too many calories, you won't have the energy you need to work out. This is one of the main reasons people quit fitness programs. They don't understand the intimate link between food and exercise. So when it's time to work out, they simply don't have the proper energy — which destroys their motivation to continue.

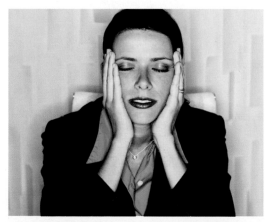

▷ Eat Smart

To get in shape, you'll need to get your blood sugar levels under control by eating four to six meals per day. Each meal provides protein, a little carbohydrate and a little fat. The fat can be built into the protein or added to the meal. But don't mistake the definition of a "meal" for a six-course feast. A typical meal might be one of the following:

☑ An egg-white omelet with vegetables and oatmeal with blueberries

☑ Chicken (seasoned to taste), sweet potatoes and a large salad with oil & vinegar

☑ Cottage cheese with fruit

Four to six meals a day sounds like a lot, but the human body is always seeking to store body fat. It doesn't care that you want to lose fat. In fact, your body would prefer to keep fat in order to accomplish its number-one goal of keeping you alive in case of future famine or drought.

Always consider the body from the inside out and not the other way around. To control your blood sugar levels, eat every two to three hours. The most effective nutrient ratios help control blood sugar to help you lose body fat.

Think ahead and prepare meals beforehand. Buy a small cooler and place some healthy snacks in it when you know you'll be out of the house for long periods of time.

▷ Premium Fuel

This doesn't have to be a massive exercise in self-denial where you eat the most boring, tasteless foods on the planet. Good fuel is important to increase performance and fitness. At the most basic level, your engine won't run without gas in the tank, and if the fuel is of poor quality, you may get started, but it's going to be rough going. And when you're running on empty, you're not going to finish the race.

You need about 64 ounces of fluid replenishment daily.

Reducing calories, increasing exercise or both can accomplish weight loss. Exercise helps weight loss by burning more calories, and building lean muscle helps increase your metabolic rate, which helps you maintain weight loss. When you increase activity, unless you make some strategic changes in your diet, you could wind up hungry all the time, which is counterproductive to your goals of weight loss and increased fitness. For optimal performance, your diet should be comprised of smaller, more frequent meals. Balance your meals with lean protein, unrefined carbohydrates from whole grains, fruits and vegetables, and healthy fats from olive oil, avocados and fatty fish. Fuel your workout with balanced snacks; following your workout, have a small, balanced snack as well. If you lose weight too quickly, that means you're not taking in enough calories.

It's unlikely you'll lose body fat by consuming 70 to 80 percent of your calories from carbohydrates. Ratios can vary quite a bit, but consuming more than 55 percent of your calories from carbohydrates will not be optimal for fat loss. Many people do quite well on extremely low-carbohydrate plans. Others do well on more moderate plans. As long as no more than 55 percent of your calories come from carbohydrates, you'll be at a good starting point.

Hydration is also critical to good physical

performance. Most people don't drink enough water to replenish what's lost daily through perspiration, urination and breathing. In cool weather, you need about 64 ounces of fluid replenishment daily, and more in the summer. Dehydration is often mistaken for fatigue, so stay hydrated and stay healthy.

If you're working out efficiently and you're maintaining a slight caloric deficit, you can actually lose up to 1.5 pounds per week. That's a lot of fat loss in the course of one year.

▷ Get Your Engine Started

Even if you haven't been consistent, the following metabolism-boosting tips should help ignite some good, steady fat loss.

☑ **Eat breakfast.** Although it may be obvious that a nutritious breakfast is important, the numberpeople who think they're doing the right thing by skipping breakfast is amazing. Think of the body from the inside out. The human body's main goal is survival. If it senses any type of emergency, it will do everything in its power to keep you alive. If you sleep through the night, then deprive the body of food in the morning, the body senses a potential famine and holds onto stored body fat to keep you alive. Remember, calories from food represent heat. Use that heat to rev up your metabolism.

☑ **Cycle calories.** For three days, consume your minimum calorie requirement based on your height, weight and goals. Then, on day four, increase your calories by an extra 400 calories (nutritious foods only). For example, if you're losing fat by consuming 1,200 calories per day, simply raise your calories to 1,600 on day four. This technique can actually get the metabolism racing and stimulate additional fat loss. Just remember that the additional calories must come from good sources of protein,

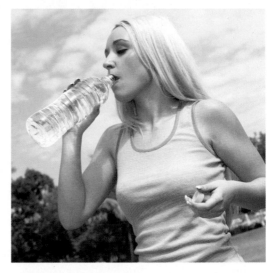

carbohydrates and fats — not junk food.

☑ **Water, water everywhere.** Muscles and other body tissues are made up of about 80 percent water. If you limit your water intake, the body will retain water and make you feel bloated. We all know how absolutely awful it feels to be bloated. It doesn't take much to retain water — the body only needs to be dehydrated by approximately 2 percent for water rentention to occur. How much should you drink? Multiply your body weight by .55 to determine how many ounces of water you need per day. By staying hydrated, you will release some excess water trapped in the body and most likely reduce your weight by a few pounds.

☑ **Drink green tea.** Green tea is a popular tea native to Japan that has many health benefits, including weight loss. It's not 100 percent certain how green tea helps with fat loss, but it appears to increase the amount of calories the body burns — not necessarily because of the small amounts of caffeine it contains, but due to a compound it contains which is abbreviated as EGCG. When purchasing green tea, make sure that the label shows that the green tea product is standardized for caffeine and EGCG.

Top 10 Fitness
Resolutions

To promise not to do a thing is the surest way to make a body go and do that very thing.

— Mark Twain, *The Adventures of Tom Sawyer*

Are you so determined to stick with your weight loss and fitness resolutions that you write them down ... in permanent black marker?

On January 1, you break out the celery sticks and hide the chips and cookies, determined to finally shed that spare tire. You're "good" for awhile. You cut calories and find time to exercise. But in a moment of weakness, you down a whole pint of ice cream. To make matters worse, you skip a workout or two ... or five. It's all downhill from there as you throw in the towel and resolve to try again ... next year.

▷ Make a Commitment

Are you determined to make your fitness resolutions a reality? Great! But be careful. "I've learned that nothing sets a person up for failure like an open-ended, generic fitness resolution," says eDiets' Chief Fitness Pro, Raphael Calzadilla.

Resolving to "lose weight" is just too generic. There is no plan of action or real goal to sink your teeth into.

Resolutions like, "I'm going to get in shape," or "I'm going to eat better," may make sense at the time, but they have no real game plan. What constitutes "healthier" eating or "better" shape?

If your resolutions are too vague and you don't have a plan to follow, then you won't have a blueprint for success. Having a vague idea of the direction you want to go is a plan to fail, or more simply put, a failure to plan. This year, plan to succeed, and you will.

A resolution needs to include what you will do to get in shape or eat well, like: "I will walk four mornings a week before work and replace the butter and oil in my cooking with cooking spray."

Make your resolutions measureable. Even though a resolution like, "I'm going to ride the stationary bike more often" is specific and realistic, it's hard to gauge. Does "more often" mean once a week or three times a week? How will you know that you've succeeded?

When you have a measurable goal ("I'm going to ride the bike for at least 30 minutes, three times a week."), it's much easier to assess your progress. For best results, think in numbers.

Visualize the results. How you picture yourself is a self-fulfilling prophecy. Daydream in detail with a realistic expectation of how you would like to look. If you see yourself as out of shape or overweight, you will perpetuate that image by simply believing it. Picture yourself standing tall, taking deep, cleansing breaths and confidently striding forward, strong and lean.

▷ Less Is More

Don't make too many resolutions. Having one to

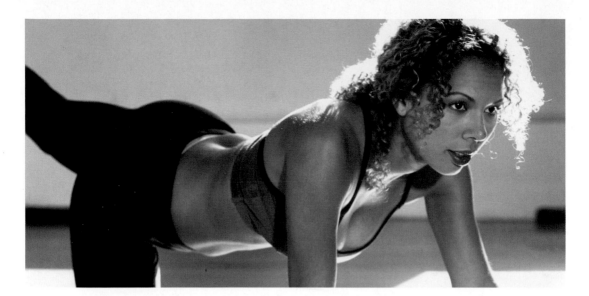

three will keep you on the right track. Plus, focusing on a few fitness goals will bring greater results than a long list that may make you feel overwhelmed. Limiting the resolutions, being focused and maintaining consistency is crucial.

Some people make so many resolutions that they can barely remember them, let alone see any through to completion. Setting only a few major goals will help you make them priorities. Write them down and tack them up on the refrigerator or the bathroom mirror, where you'll be reminded of them each day.

▷ Keep the Faith

Don't let a minor lapse stop you dead in your tracks. If you fail to work out one week, don't give up completely. Just pick up where you left off the next week or even the next day. And be patient about seeing results — losing weight and getting in shape takes time. Strengthen your resolve by deciding why weight loss is important to you and by visualizing your success at least three times a day.

Research shows you're 10 times more likely to reach your goal if you make a commitment, rather than simply having a desire to do so.

People who make resolutions and succeed in reaching their goals have the same number of slip-ups as those who resolve and fail.

This year, plan to succeed, and you will.

Don't use a short-term approach to solve a long-term problem. We secretly believe we can lose weight, get in shape and then resume all our bad habits. We fail to realize that weight management is a lifestyle challenge that requires permanent changes. Losing weight and keeping it off takes a commitment of time and energy. We have to gear up for the contest if we're going to stay on the winning track.

You will find 10 resolutions on the following page. Pick the ones that appeal to you most and fill in the blanks, or modify the resolution based on your fitness experience. Remember, don't choose all of them. Just one to three resolutions is all you need to see some success.

It's a contract of sorts. If you breach the terms, you won't be sent to the big house, but at least you will feel the commitment is a little more concrete when you see it in writing.

▷ The Contract

I hereby resolve to implement these fitness resolutions to lose weight and shape up:

1. **I will lose four pounds per month for a total of _____ pounds by _____ (date).** If you treat weight loss like a sprint, you will be back at square one in no time flat. Nutrition experts will tell you that a healthy, sustainable weight loss is about two pounds per week.

2. **For three months, I will work out three times per week for a minimum of 30 minutes. If my schedule allows, I'll add a fourth day during Month 4.** If twice per week is more realistic, go with that. The key is consistency. Do what's realistic based on your lifestyle. A little can go a long way.

3. **I will increase my endurance by two minutes per week so I can power walk an additional 16 minutes per workout session by the beginning of Month 3.** You can choose any form of cardio (jogging, Spinning, aerobics), but there must be a realistic time increase and a time frame goal.

4. **I will perform 20 minutes of resistance exercise twice per week using a whole-body workout routine.** Most commonly performed with weights, resistance training is an essential component of weight loss and muscle toning. Concentrate on proper form. Feel a little burn, and you'll be on your way.

5. **I will find a fun fitness videotape/DVD and do it twice per week for the first two months.** This resolution is great if you dislike traditional workouts. It provides a little extra guidance and can be a fun addition to a normally dull workout.

6. **I will find a group exercise class such as Spinning, kickboxing or Jazzercise.** I will sign up for the class and commit to two days per week for 30 days. Working out alone can get lonely! Odds are, you will bond with your classmates and won't want to let them down by not showing up.

7. **I will increase my flexibility by stretching three days per week for seven to 10 minutes.** Flexibility is important, and it doesn't take all that much to improve upon it. Stretching will help lengthen the muscles, while increasing blood flow and muscle temperature. This will lead to fewer injuries.

8. **I will go for two 15-minute walks per day, from Monday through Friday.** Fit in one walk at lunchtime and one walk after dinner. This fitness resolution is for those of you who are so busy you can't make it to the gym. It's also a great way to get you away from the dinner table and off the couch.

9. **I will hire a personal trainer for two sessions per week for a total of 20 sessions.** Don't worry if you think you have to commit a wad of money. This resolution is for those who need a good push and some teaching and motivation to go along with it. A fitness trainer just might be the incentive you need to work out, even on days when you don't feel like it.

10. **I will find a friend who also needs to work out.** That friend and I will commit to two months of regular exercise that adheres to at least two of the resolutions above. Two's company, and when that little devil on your shoulder tells you to bypass the gym, you'll know you have a friend waiting who you can't just ditch.

When you find the resolutions that fit you best, dig in and go for it. This is your best chance to reach your goals. While other people's resolutions may fall by the wayside, you will be well on your way to a positive lifestyle change.

Real People, Real Results.

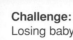

Challenge: Losing baby weight	Start Weight: 227 lbs. End Weight: 148 lbs. Pounds Lost: 79

Results not typical.

New Mom Erin Lost 79 lbs!

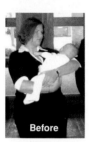

Before

When it comes to obesity, people can be cruel, mostly to themselves.

Nobody knows this better than featured dieter Erin L. This 27-year-old Texan used to look at herself in the mirror and say "mooooo." Erin — who is 5 feet, 8 inches tall — says dragging around 227 pounds made her feel like "a cow put out to pasture." She despised going out in public, and she found the attitudes of her family and friends changed along with her waistline.

But it didn't take a cattle prod to jolt her into action. Erin found all the motivation she needed with the eDiets.com Weight-Loss Plan, which helped her drop a beefy 79 pounds. Today, the stunning stay-at-home mom weighs just 148 pounds and is in the best shape of her life. But she doesn't only measure her success in pounds lost. She's also trimmed 50 inches from her chest, waist, belly, hips, legs and arms combined. And her body fat has shrunk from 39.3 percent to 21.8 percent.

Making such a dramatic transformation was no small feat. Before eDiets, Erin had tried everything from fad diets to pills. While she would lose a few pounds here and there, nothing could offset the weight gain caused by a prescription drug.

Born and raised in south Louisiana, she loves Cajun cooking — gumbo, red beans and rice, Boudin sausage and crawfish etouffee.

A few months after giving birth to her son, Nathan, Erin's weight loss slowed. Stuck at 227 pounds, she turned to eDiets and took it one step at a time. She felt she first needed to control her overeating, and the awesome eDiets recipes made it easy. She never felt deprived — especially when she indulged in a weekly treat.

"When I first started eDiets, I became addicted to the waffles with ricotta cheese and fruit cocktail. I still eat that. There are a lot of great recipes. When I need something different, I know I can go to eDiets and look for a new dish."

Exercise, of course, was a key component of her weight loss. Even though she has Nathan and her stepson Christopher to take care of, she always makes time for working out. She planned her workouts a month ahead of time, using the gym's childcare center. Erin loves exercise so much that she is working toward getting certified as a personal trainer so she can help others.

Test Your **Fitness Savvy**

One of the problems in our society is that we simply assume the concepts, products and methods we see on TV will work.

It's important not only to ask, "What is my goal?" but also, "Will this work?" "Does it make sense?" and, "Is it safe?" These are all smart questions that should be asked before you spend your cash on a nifty-looking gadget that will most likely end up collecting dust in your bedroom.

Fitness savvy doesn't require a degree in biochemistry or exercise physiology, just a little knowledge about the human body.

"A lot of diet books and supplement companies have only one thing in mind — profits," says eDiets' Chief Fitness Pro Raphael Calzadilla. "Profit is a great thing, but not at the expense of people who are searching for a way to get lean and healthy."

With so much conflicting information about what it takes to lose weight and stay in shape, Calzadilla doesn't blame consumers for being confused. In fact, he says that the American Council on Exercise (ACE) asked its trainer base to conduct a poll of their clients to uncover the most common fitness myths that confuse people. Many believed the following statements to be true. Let's find out.

☑ **Women Who Lift Weights Will Get Bulky Muscles.**

Myth. "A woman has one-third the testosterone of a man, so putting on a ton of muscle is not going to happen," Calzadilla says. "You'll look bulky if you're carrying excessive body fat and building muscle. But if you're reducing body fat, you will eventually see those lean, defined muscles."

☑ **Spot Reducing Is Possible.**

Myth. The human body loses fat in different places at different rates. "It's impossible to spot reduce. Generally, the first place you gain fat is the last place you lose it."

☑ **No Pain, No Gain.**

Myth. "There is absolutely no reason to cause pain in the gym," Calzadilla says. Natural progression is a good way to ensure progress, with slow, systematic increases in the amount of weight you lift, gradual increases in cardiovascular endurance and slow, steady flexibility progression.

☑ **Exercise Requires a Hefty Time Commitment.**

Myth. Calzadilla says, "Consistency and level of effort is the key. I'd rather see someone work out three days per week with enthusiasm and intensity than five inconsistent days of lackadaisical effort."

☑ **If You Exercise, You Can Eat Whatever You Want.**

Myth. "Today's big message in the world of nutrition and personal training is that most people need to eat more to stimulate the metabolism," Calzadilla says. "The truth is, you need the correct amount of total calories to lose body fat. Exercising will burn calories, but if you're eating anything you want and are over maintenance calories, you'll most likely gain fat."

☑ **There's a Quick Fix Out There.**

Myth. "There is no best and only way to work out," Raphael says. "In reality, it's all good if it works for you, but you don't want to stay with any of it for too long. The body will adapt to any exercise routine in approximately four to six weeks. Vary volume of sets, time between sets, reps, exercises, cardiovascular exercises and exercise tapes. Manipulate your routine every three to four weeks and view change as the key constant."

▷ Doing It Right

Most workout blunders stem from a lack of knowledge or misinformation. Here are some tips for avoiding the most common mistakes.

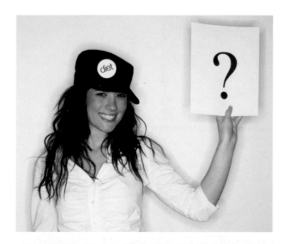

Believing that eating a little less and going on a diet will get the results you seek.

Total calories are important, but so are the amounts of protein, carbohydrates and fats in the diet. A slight caloric deficit (less than maintenance) must be adhered to as well as eating small meals and snacks every two to three hours to control blood sugar. Blood-sugar control will help you to lose fat.

Expecting perfection from your nutrition program all the time.

Most of us love food and need to find a way to enjoy a modest amount of treats. Giving up the special foods you enjoy can lead to frustration and cheating, so moderation is key. Adding a sensible amount of treats into your diet is the best way to stay on plan.

Performing countless abdominal crunches will get rid of the "pouch" area on the lower tummy.

Crunches only strengthen muscle. They won't flatten the stomach. Just as 200 bicep curls will not make the arm smaller, 200 abdominal crunches will not reduce your waist.

Not having a realistic workout schedule that fits into your lifestyle.

"You need a plan that's based on the way you live your life," Calzadilla says. If your plan has you working out five to six days per week with little spare time, you need a more sensible approach. Try starting with two workouts per week and increasing to three workouts in the third or fourth week.

If you're determined enough to dedicate your time and energy to getting in shape, it would be a shame if you were to make the effort in vain. Let's put your motivation to good use!

▷ True or False?

1. **Lifting lighter weights will make your muscles more defined and cut.**

2. **A lot of cardio is the most efficient way to lose body fat.**

3. **You can gain 20 pounds of muscle in a few months.**

4. **The best way to lose fat is to eat very few calories.**

5. **The best way to lose fat is to eat a lot of calories.**

6. **Calories are the only things that count when trying to lose fat or gain muscle.**

7. **A woman will get "manly" muscles if she lifts heavier weight.**

8. **One pound of muscle and one pound of fat are the same size.**

9. **You can put on a lot of muscle and lose a lot of fat at the same time.**

10. **The more protein you consume, the more muscle you'll add to your body.**

Answers

1. FALSE! Reduced body fat creates the "cut" look, not high (15 or more) reps. Reduced body fat is a result of efficient weight training, cardiovascular exercise and nutrition that places you in somewhat of a calorie deficit.

2. FALSE! Excessive cardio strips muscle mass and body fat. For each pound of muscle you add, you'll burn up to 50 additional calories per day. Stripping muscle mass will sabotage your efforts.

3. FALSE! Claims that a routine or supplement can help you gain "10 pounds of muscle in a month" are marketing scams. It takes diligent weight training with sufficient overload and consistency to build muscle mass. Except for initial muscular gains, it can take up to a year to gain five to six pounds of muscle mass.

4. FALSE! If you eat very little, the body will hold on to stored body fat.

5. FALSE! Most people need to eat more to stimulate their metabolism. The truth is, you need the correct amount of total calories to lose body fat, not simply more food.

6. FALSE! A balance of protein, carbohydrates and fats is the most efficient way to lose fat and gain muscle. The key to losing fat and gaining muscle is controlling and manipulating insulin levels. Excessive spikes in blood sugar will put you at risk for diabetes and your body will hold on to stored fat.

7. FALSE! This myth never seems to die. Unless she is on anabolic steroids, growth hormones or other chemicals, a woman will never achieve the muscular size of a man.

8. FALSE! One pound of muscle and one pound of fat weigh the same. The difference is in total volume. A pound of muscle is about the size of a baseball; a pound of fat is three times the size and looks like wiggly gelatin.

9. FALSE! You can put on muscle and lose some fat, but the body functions best when it has one goal at a time. If your goal is to put on a lot of muscle, make that your main objective. If your goal is to lose significant body fat, focus on preserving your hard-earned muscle mass.

10. FALSE! The body requires the right amount of protein to put on muscle. A weight trainer requires a lot more protein than the sedentary person. The body uses protein, carbohydrates and a small amount of fat to build muscle.

Real People, Real Results.

Challenge: Sticking with a program	Start Weight: 215 lbs. End Weight: 162 lbs. Pounds Lost: 53

Results not typical.

Victoria Lost 53 lbs. Eating Six Times a Day!

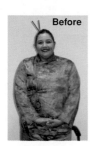
Before

Victoria V. can best be described as a victorious quitter. Since signing up for eDiets' Glycemic Impact Diet and losing 53 pounds, she has quit smoking, stopped getting sick and quit wearing size-16 clothes.

Today, the 5-foot 6-inch Floridian enjoys her sleek new figure. Her energy has skyrocketed, and her body, which transformed from 215 pounds to an incredible 162 pounds, is healthier than ever.

"I can get out there and do some amazing physical things that I never thought I could do before, and it's just amazing," Victoria says. "Yeah, my life has changed."

The former dancer's weight struggle began when her intensely active lifestyle changed.

The 33-year-old went from being a dancing diva on her toes 10 hours a day to sitting behind a desk, lucky to get four hours of exercise a week. And she continued eating as if she was getting 10 hours of exercise a day. She hardly recognized herself in the mirror.

"I was still eating pasta three times a week and starches and rice, and my body reacted to that, and I just ballooned up. I hated the feeling. I would get out of breath. I had never been like that before."

Bent on getting her life back in shape, she took her sister's advice and checked out what eDiets had to offer and found the GI Diet.

Victoria had no problem adjusting to her new plan. Low glycemic-impact foods helped sustain her energy throughout the day without the swings she endured from caffeine and hunger.

She was able to control her carbohydrate cravings but liked that she didn't have to give them up completely. Victoria also loved that there were no special foods involved and that she was able to eat several times a day. She never felt deprived.

The fit and firm Floridian is dancing again and is enjoying Pilates and Spinning classes.

Victoria is only 15 pounds away from her goal weight. She continues using eDiets to maintain her new healthy lifestyle.

"At first, I didn't know if I would be able to stick to it over long periods of time. It's been two years, and not only have I been able to stick to it, but I actually look forward to creating my menus. If I hadn't given it that one month or that first six months, I never would have known that I could do it myself."

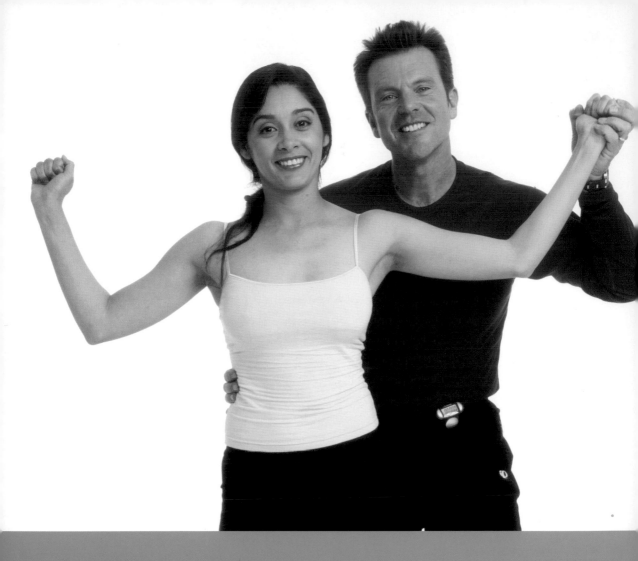

Expert Advice

The advice and instruction of a personal trainer is ideal for learning proper form, efficiency and injury prevention.

Bob Greene,
Celebrity Trainer

The name Bob Greene should sound familiar. You've seen him on *The Oprah Winfrey Show*, *The TODAY Show*, *Good Morning America* and E! Bob has been Oprah's personal trainer for more than 10 years, and he helped the Queen of Daytime TV get into the best shape of her life.

But Bob isn't simply a flashy celebrity trainer without credentials. He studied health and physical education at the University of Delaware, then completed his master's degree in exercise physiology at the University of Arizona. He is an exercise physiologist, a certified personal trainer and a member of both the American College of Sports Medicine and the American Council on Exercise. Greene has specialized in metabolism, fitness, and weight loss for the past 20 years.

▷ Make Yourself Over

Bob Greene's Total Body Makeover is a 12-week plan that's great for beginners who don't know where to start an exercise program. It includes functional, cardiovascular and strength exercises.

"These three components determine whether or not you are 'officially' fit. There are certainly many people who possess high levels of all three types of fitness, but more often, people are 'fit' in one or two areas and are completely unfit in the others," Greene says.

☑ **Functional exercises** comprise flexibility exercises, abdominal crunches, back and shoulder exercises, and lower-leg exercises which can be done in only eight to 10 minutes.

☑ **Cardiovascular exercise** refers to the ability of the heart, lungs and arteries to deliver oxygen to working muscles, and to the muscles' ability to use that oxygen for work over a sustained period of time. Cardiovascular fitness increases the rate at which the body burns calories.

What you are doing during an aerobic workout is modestly starving your body of oxygen. This sends a message to your heart and lungs that they must become stronger (just as other muscles in your body become stronger when you train with weights), and tells your muscles that they need to manufacture more aerobic enzymes so that they can process more oxygen.

Your body responds by strengthening all these systems. But these results are contingent upon depriving (only slightly) the body of oxygen while exercising.

To continue to improve, you must continue to challenge your body aerobically on a regular basis. Just test your capabilities   don't overexert yourself.

Cardio shouldn't involve pain or require a great investment of time. Walking at a brisk pace (a 15-minute mile or 4 mph) burns almost as many calories as jogging for the same distance. When you jog, you can cover the same distance more quickly, but it may be too strenuous for some.

☑ **Strength training** acts as the primary calorie burner by boosting your metabolism. "It will strengthen your body and allow it to function more efficiently so you can perform your aerobic exercise at higher levels, which will decrease your percentage of body fat and tone muscles," Greene says.

Another important, yet often overlooked, benefit of strength training is the way it combats two of the most profound effects of aging: the loss of muscle and the loss of bone mass (osteoporosis).

Get creative. The resistance of water is perfect for a strength-training workout. Instead of weights, the water itself provides the resistance. One of the easiest ways to create resistance in the water is to cup your hands and push or pull the water away from you. Other devices, such as hand-held paddles and water chutes, can increase the resistance to intensify the workout.

▷ Getting Started

"Committing is the first step, but many other steps must follow. Change is a progression, and each bit of forward momentum you make will give you confidence to take on the next challenge. You will experience a series of accomplishments – some big, some small, but each one important. Improving yourself is like building a house. You need to set down a

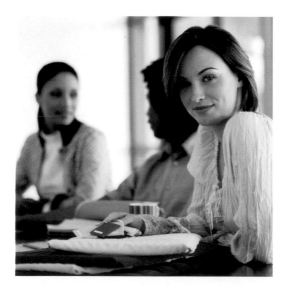

strong foundation (your commitment to yourself), then layer on it, floor by floor, room by room," Greene says.

There's a logical progression to the building process. Once you shore up your emotional foundation — that is, your commitment, self-control and a truthful understanding of yourself — you need to find a way to put exercise into your life on a regular basis. The third step is to improve your diet by tossing out all the foods you know aren't on the program and replacing them with healthier choices.

Most people do not follow this progression. Don't make the mistake they do and begin with a diet then cut calories. When you do this, you lower your metabolism (the rate at which you burn calories). But if you start by exercising, you raise your metabolism. In addition, exercise can provide you with a powerful incentive to eat well. When you exercise, you'll see changes in your body that, hopefully, will inspire you to eat more healthfully.

That's absolutely essential. Plus, if you're not eating nutritiously, you'll really feel it when you work out — it'll be hard to keep your energy up. Get in the exercise habit before you start tinkering with your diet, and you'll keep your metabolism going strong so your new eating habits can immediately yield positive results.

"There's no single secret to getting a better body. It's essential to examine your whole life. Powerful change occurs by taking small steps toward your goal every day of your life. We all have setbacks. You'll have bad days and good — but if you're committed, I know you'll succeed," Greene says.

Take a closer look at some of the other benefits Total Body Makeover has to offer:

It's a non-intimidating, easy-to-follow 12-week program. For example, cardiovascular exercises build to a total of 60 minutes in week 1, then you add five minutes per week. By week 12, you're comfortably performing a minimum of 115 minutes of cardiovascular exercise per week.

The gradual progression of exercises during the 12-week period trains the body to handle additional exercise capacity. This gradual progression is the key to forming lifelong exercise habits.

> ## "If you're committed to your own well-being, I know you'll succeed."

It provides a guideline for the most efficient cardio exercises to the least efficient. Participants can then make smart choices that will increase their rate of calorie-burning exercises.

In later weeks, strength training with dumbbells is added to the program, which provides for a natural progression – the key to preventing injury and adhering to the program.

Animations and descriptions of each strength-training exercise are provided on eDiets.com to teach you proper exercise form.

The program can be done in the comfort of your home or in a gym. But keep a few things in mind if you choose to work out at a gym. There are a variety of places you can go to exercise, but finding one that fits all of your needs can sometimes be a chore. Keep in mind that whatever your specific needs and interests are, you should be able to get to your facility within a 10- to 15-minute drive from where you live or work — a longer commute will likely cut down on how many times a week you exercise and/or how long you actually work out.

Different types of facilities specialize in certain kinds of exercise and cater to a specific clientele. If this is not evident during your initial tour, ask to have a complimentary workout — some places will give you a free trial week. Just be sure you like the place you are joining.

TOTAL BODY MAKEOVER
from Oprah's Trainer, BOB GREENE

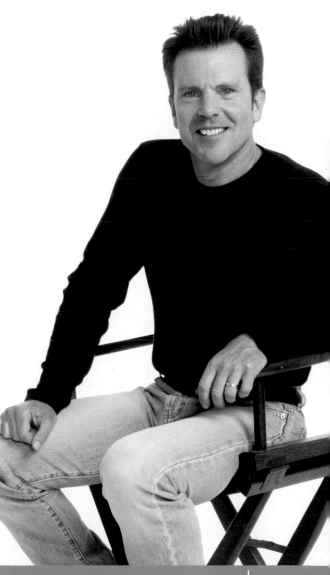

Bill Phillips'
5 Tips for a Flatter Tummy

Bill Phillips'
Eating
for Life Plan™

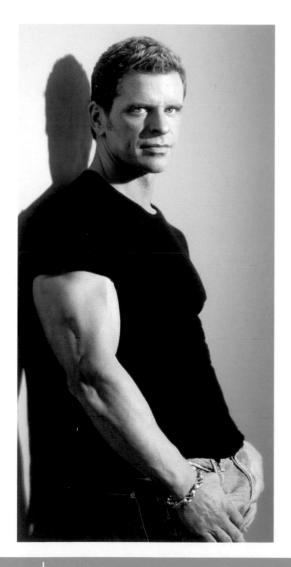

All the sit-ups in the world won't help you achieve a tighter stomach if you don't have the one-two punch of healthy eating and exercise. Nobody knows this better than fitness guru Bill Phillips.

The founder of the Body for Life program and the follow-up diet plan, Eating for Life, says far too many people overlook the importance of a good nutrition plan. Little do they know, it's an integral part of the weight-loss equation. Phillips shares the secrets behind an effective eating regimen and a balanced fitness program.

▷ The Big Four

The Eating for Life Plan is based on four primary ingredients: the Right Foods, the Right Amounts, the Right Combos and the Right Times. When you combine these four ingredients, you will have the Right Recipe to feed your body in a balanced, healthy, hearty, satisfying and effective way. You'll increase energy, build strength, look and feel younger, and lose body fat.

The goal of Phillips' Eating for Life plan is to help you lose weight, feel great and not feel hungry. To keep your body working at peak performance, you need balance. The plan eliminates instability and provides the foods that work best for you. Phillips provides guidelines on everything from managing your kitchen to streamlining your grocery shopping.

But this plan isn't about deprivation. Phillips describes his approach as "basic and balanced with no obscure foods." He is determined to destruct the myth that "healthy food" is boring.

"I'm telling you, loud and clear, here and now, that you can and should look forward to a lifetime of enjoying food that is both nutritious and delicious," Phillips says. "That's a fact."

The Eating for Life plan can even be customized to your tastes. After all, Phillips knows that when it comes to preferences, one size does not fit all. He says it's time to take back what's rightfully yours —enjoyment in eating.

"People need to look at becoming healthy and fit instead of just losing weight."

"When you're planning, you're being proactive, not reactive. The downside of being reactive is that there are so many temptations, so many unhealthy things to eat in the current environment that you really have to put yourself in the position to do the right thing," he says. "When you're reacting in the wrong situation, it's hard to do the right thing. By planning, you can create the right situation and set the table for your success."

▷ Satisfy Your Appetite

According to Phillips, too many people are stuffing themselves with food, yet starving for proper nutrition. It's only when the body receives the nutrients it craves that you'll start to satisfy your appetite, he says.

"Eating for Life is very intuitive. It works with your body, not against it. After a few weeks getting the hang of it, it really feels right. Common sense gives you an intuitive feeling that you're on the right path," Phillips says.

"For long-term success, this is very important because you have to feel right about what you're doing. The science behind Eating for Life is also important because if you know that you're feeding yourself in a way that's consistent with what scientific studies supported, you feel confident, and this helps with long-term success."

Although healthy eating is the core of Phillips' Eating for Life program, regular exercise is just as important. While some people would have you believe that food and fitness are natural-born enemies, Phillips says the two are absolutely inseparable. In fact, food and fitness are two of his greatest passions. According to Phillips, you can "indulge your love for food and feed your fondness for fitness." Exercise doesn't just help burn calories; it also redirects the body's cravings. Adopting a regular exercise program will even help you to control your appetite.

▷ Listen To Your Body

Eating for Life is about listening to your body. It follows the concept that your body was built to move. Once you start exercising, Phillips says you will automatically hunger for the nutrient-rich foods your body needs for fuel.

"Exercise is scientifically proven to help people break the pattern of addictive cravings for unhealthy foods. One of the reasons I so enthusiastically encourage exercise as a way of helping people change their eating habits is because it also soothes what the brain is craving. People who have struggled with making changes in their diet know all too well that those cravings are coming from the mind. The body doesn't crave anything. Working with the brain chemistry through exercise is an important part of success," Phillips says.

Research has shown that participating in regular exercise increases your body's beta endorphin levels. The more of these neurotransmitters you have, the easier it is for you to stay in a good mood and control your cravings for food. Phillips stresses that healthy eating and exercise pack a powerful one-two punch. You really can't have one without the other when you're working toward a toned body.

Exercise increases your body's need for nutrients. Exercising a nutrient-deficient body actually creates worse nutrient deficiencies. For exercise to be effective and for it to help improve your health, you must feed your body plenty of protein, vitamins, minerals, essential fats, quality carbohydrates and drink ample amounts of water. Then you'll be able to build a stronger, healthier, leaner, better and more energetic body with each workout.

Everyone has the right genetics to be in great shape.

"People need to look at becoming healthy and fit instead of just losing weight," Phillips says. "Your aspiration should be making your body fit, strong and energetic instead of smaller."

Don't believe the myth that you need to have a certain type of genetics to lose weight and be fit. According to Phillips, everyone has the right genetics to be in great shape.

"Eating for Life produces predictable results in virtually every healthy adult," Phillips says. "Recent scientific discoveries in gene mapping show that you and I are 99 percent identical in terms of our genetic fingerprint. And while that one percent difference is conspicuous (height, hair color, eye color, etc.), it does not mean that each person responds completely differently to proper nutrition and regular exercise."

▷ Let's Get Started

If you've lost your resolve and found a few more pounds along the way, it may be time to belly up to a brand-new workout regimen. It may have been a shortage of proper knowledge about fitness and nutrition that led to your past diet's demise, but now is the perfect time to get back on track. With the right eating and exercise regimen — and 5 great tips from a prominent fitness expert — you'll start seeing results fast.

▷ Tummy-Trimming

1. When you eat smaller, more balanced portions of food, you significantly change the way the belly looks. One of the reasons that doing 100 sit-ups never results in a flat belly is because the gut is too full. By eating smaller portions, you're moving toward a flatter belly.

2. Overall body fat contributes to how lean the belly is. The body's fat compartment is one system. Doing leg exercises actually burns five times more body fat than doing sit-ups. Exercising the whole body is the way to burn fat off the belly. The notion that sit-ups burn fat off the belly is a myth.

3. Exercising the ab muscles twice a week is plenty. Muscles become stronger and firmer through adaptation. You stress the muscle, then it recovers and comes back stronger and better. Muscles need ample time to recover.

4. Most people don't realize that their posture affects the tightness of their abdominal muscles. Weak abs cause you to lean forward and for your shoulders to sag. Practice healthy posture by keeping your shoulders up and back straight while walking, sitting at your desk and exercising. Proper exercise posture helps flatten the belly as well.

5. Two highly effective ab exercises are crunches and stability ball leg lifts. These exercises work the most muscle fibers and get the best results the fastest. The stability ball causes you to use virtually every muscle in the upper and lower abs. The whole midsection core has to work to pull off the crunches and leg lifts.

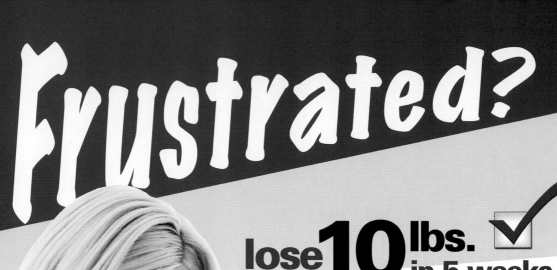

Frustrated?

lose 10 lbs. ✓
in 5 weeks

Have you outgrown your "skinny jeans"? Then get the skinny on the **eDiets® Weight Loss Plan**. It's personalized for the way you live and the way you like to eat, so it's always a perfect fit.

Try It On For Size!

Log on to www.eDiets.com

eDiets.com®
WEIGHT-LOSS PLAN

© 2006 eDiets.com, Inc. eDiets and eDiets.com are registered trademarks of eDiets.com, Inc. All rights reserved.

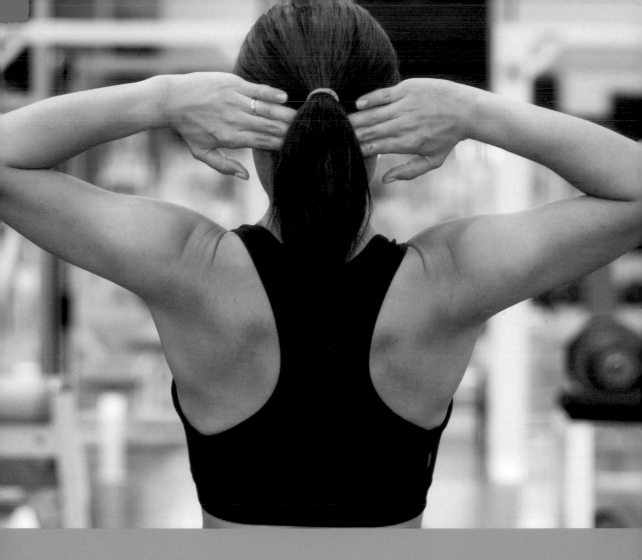

The Right **Moves**

Target your body's trouble spots with the best toning exercises. As with all workouts, do your best to follow the proper format.

THE INNER-THIGH SPECIALTY WORKOUT

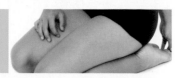

Fitness-Band Standing Leg Adduction

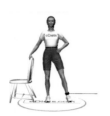
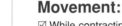
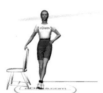
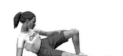

Starting Position:
☑ Attach a fitness band to a door at ankle height (the band should come with a door attachment).
☑ Attach the fitness band to your left ankle.
☑ Stand with your left side facing the door with your weight on the right leg and your right hand on a chair or table to balance your body.
☑ Place your left hand on your hip.
☑ Maintain a slight bend in the knees throughout the exercise.

Movement:
☑ While contracting the inner thigh muscles (adductors), move the left leg past the right leg, stopping when you feel a contraction in the inner thigh.
☑ Slowly return to the starting position.
☑ After the set, perform the movement with the other leg.

Key Points:
☑ Exhale while moving the leg across the body.
☑ Inhale when returning to the starting position.
☑ Perform 15 slow and controlled repetitions for each leg and then immediately go to the next exercise.

Fitness-Band Standing Leg Adduction

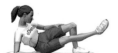

Starting Position:
☑ Lie on your right side with your right arm supporting your upper body.
☑ Your right leg should be straight, and your left leg should be bent with your foot on the floor.
☑ Support your weight on your right arm and left leg.

Movement:
☑ While keeping the inner thigh muscles tight, lift your right leg up until you feel a contraction of the inner thigh muscles.
☑ After completing the set on the right side, perform the exercise on the left side.

Key Points:
☑ Exhale while lifting your leg up.
☑ Inhale when returning to the starting position.
☑ You may use ankle weights to increase the level of difficulty.
☑ If you are an intermediate exerciser, you can add resistance to the inner thigh as you are lifting. You can resist your inner thigh with your hand or use a weighted object.
☑ Perform 20 slow and controlled repetitions on each side and immediately go to the next exercise.

Starting Position:

☑ Place an ankle weight on your left ankle.
☑ Stand erect with your weight on the right leg with a soft bend in the knee and your right hand on a chair or table for balance.
☑ Place your left hand on your hip.

Movement:

☑ While contracting the inner thigh muscles, move your left leg past your right leg.
☑ Slowly return to the starting position. Stop when the left leg is in front of the right leg.

Key Points:

☑ Exhale while lifting the weight.
☑ Inhale when returning to the starting position.
☑ If you have one dominant leg, start with the less dominant leg first.
☑ Perform 15 to 20 slow and controlled repetitions.
☑ After completing the routine, take a 60-second break and repeat the above sequence two additional times – this is the ultimate goal.
☑ Beginners should perform one set, intermediates two sets and advanced exercisers three sets. Just remember to focus all your attention on the inner thighs and perform the movements with perfect form.

THREE GREAT TUMMY-TIGHTENING EXERCISES

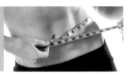

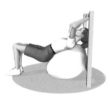

Starting Position:

☑ Lie on the ball with your upper back supported by the ball and hands above your head holding onto a solid support such as the support for a cable machine in the gym or the footboard of your bed at home.
☑ Bring your legs up until your hips and knees are each at a 90-degree angle.

Movement:

☑ Contracting the abdominals, curl your legs up toward your body.
☑ Slowly return to the starting position.

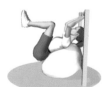

Key Points:

☑ Exhale while lifting your legs.
☑ Inhale while returning to the starting position.
☑ Lower your legs only as far as you can while maintaining control.

Two-Leg Bent Knee Raise

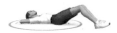

Starting Position:
☑ Lie on the floor with both hands behind your head.
☑ Bend your knees at a 90-degree angle.

Movement:
☑ Contracting your abdominals, raise both legs maintaining the angle at the knees.
☑ Slowly return to the starting position stopping just short of your feet touching the floor.

Key Points:
☑ Exhale while raising your legs.
☑ Inhale while returning to the starting position.
☑ This exercise should not be performed if you have a weak lower back or any discomfort is felt in the back.

Oblique Sit-Up

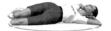

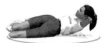

Starting Position:
☑ Lie on the floor with your knees bent to the right side.
☑ Place your hands lightly behind your head.

Movement:
☑ Contracting the obliques, lift your shoulders off the floor toward the left side until your obliques fully contract.
☑ Slowly return to the starting position stopping just short of your shoulders touching the floor.
☑ After completing the set on one side, repeat on the other.

Key Points:
☑ Exhale while contracting the obliques.
☑ Inhale while returning to the starting position.
☑ Be sure to keep your head and neck relaxed.
☑ Keep your eyes focused on the ceiling to avoid leading with your chin.
☑ You must hold the contraction very tightly for at least 40 seconds. If you can't hold the contraction for 40 seconds, keep practicing, and your time eventually will improve.

Barbell Rear Squat

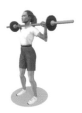

Starting Position:

☑ Place the barbell across the back of your shoulders. Be sure it is not resting on your neck.
☑ Place feet flat on the floor, shoulder width apart.

Movement:

☑ Concentrating on the butt, lower your body by bending from your hips and knees, stopping when your thighs are parallel with the floor.
☑ Slowly return to the starting position.

Key Points:

☑ Inhale as you lower your body.
☑ Exhale while returning to the starting position.
☑ Do not let your knees ride over your toes (you should be able to see your feet at all times).
☑ It helps to find a marker on the wall to keep your eye on as you lift and lower; otherwise, your head may tend to fall forward, and your body will follow.
☑ Think about sitting back in a chair as you are lowering down.
☑ Push off with your heels as you return to the starting position.
☑ Perform 20 slow and controlled repetitions and immediately go to the next exercise.
☑ You may want to try this exercise without weights until you master the movement. It is a very effective exercise that involves most of the muscle groups of the lower body, but if done improperly, it can lead to injuries.

Straight Leg Reverse Lift

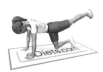

Starting Position:

☑ Start this exercise on your hands and knees.
☑ Straighten your left leg as if you were going to do a push-up.
☑ Keep the right leg bent, supporting your weight along with your arms.

Movement:

☑ Contracting the buttocks muscles, lift your left leg up toward the ceiling, stopping when you feel a full contraction of the buttocks.
☑ Slowly return to the starting position.
☑ After completing the set on the left side, repeat on the right side.

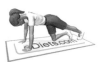

Key Points:

☑ Exhale while lifting the leg.
☑ Inhale while returning to the starting position.
☑ Perform 20 repetitions on each side and immediately go to the next exercise.
☑ Do not let the back arch.
☑ If you are an intermediate or advanced exerciser, you can add an ankle weight to the working leg to make it more challenging.

Bent-Leg Reverse Kick-Up

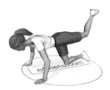

Starting Position:
☑ Start this exercise on your hands and knees on a mat.

Movement:
☑ Raise your left leg up until it is parallel with the floor with a slight bend in the knee. Support your weight with your arms and right leg.
☑ While contracting the butt, lift your left leg up and toward the ceiling, maintaining a bend in the knee.
☑ Slowly return to the starting position.
☑ After completing the set on the left side, repeat on the right side.

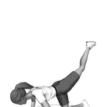

Key Points:
☑ Raise your left leg up until it is parallel with the floor with a slight bend in the knee. Support your weight with your arms and right leg.
☑ While contracting the butt, lift your left leg up and toward the ceiling, maintaining a bend in the knee.
☑ Slowly return to the starting position.
☑ After completing the set on the left side, repeat on the right side.

REDUCE UGLY BACK FLAB

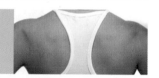

Cable Two-Arm Lat Pulldown

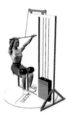

Starting Position:
☑ Extend your arms up and reach for a straight bar with an overhand grip.
☑ Sit tall with your knees supported under the leg pad, with the knees and hips at a 90-degree angle.
☑ Arms should be wider than shoulder-width apart with a slight bend in the elbows.
☑ Relax your shoulders and keep your chest lifted.

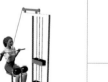

Movement:
☑ While contracting the upper back muscles, pull the bar down, leading with the elbows and stopping when the bar is just above your chest.
☑ Slowly return to the starting position, stopping just short of the weight stack touching.

Key Points:
☑ While contracting the upper back muscles, pull the bar down, leading with the elbows and stopping when the bar is just above your chest.
☑ Slowly return to the starting position, stopping just short of the weight stack touching.

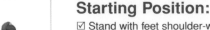

Dumbbell Bent-Over Row

Starting Position:

☑ Stand with feet shoulder-width apart and a slight bend in the knees.
☑ Hold a dumbbell in each hand and bend forward from the hips until the upper body is at about 45 degrees.
☑ Extend the arms down, keeping your shoulder blades together.

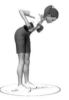

Movement:

☑ Stand with feet shoulder-width apart and a slight bend in the knees.
☑ Hold a dumbbell in each hand and bend forward from the hips until the upper body is at about 45 degrees.
☑ Extend the arms down, keeping your shoulder blades together.

Key Points:

☑ Stand with feet shoulder-width apart and a slight bend in the knees.
☑ Hold a dumbbell in each hand and bend forward from the hips until the upper body is at about 45 degrees.
☑ Extend the arms down, keeping your shoulder blades together.

Fitball Prone Trunk Extension

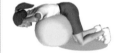

Starting Position:

☑ Lie on the ball with your knees on the floor and feet up on the toes.
☑ Place your fingertips gently on the sides of your head.
☑ Maintain a neutral spine, with head and neck relaxed as a natural extension of the spine.

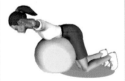

Movement:

☑ Lie on the ball with your knees on the floor and feet up on the toes.
☑ Place your fingertips gently on the sides of your head.
☑ Maintain a neutral spine, with head and neck relaxed as a natural extension of the spine.

Key Points:

☑ Exhale while lifting your body.
☑ Inhale when returning to the starting position.
☑ Do not hyperextend your back and/or overdo the range of motion.
☑ Attempt one to three sets of each exercise for 10 to 12 repetitions on alternate days of the week and focus on precise form at all times.

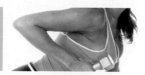

Fitball Triceps Dips

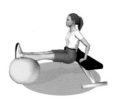

Starting Position:
☑ Sit on a bench with palms down and fingers grasping the edge of bench.
☑ Place both heels on the ball.
☑ Slide your body off the bench balancing between your hands and feet.
☑ Keep movement very controlled. Keep feet together and legs straight with a slight bend in the knees..

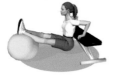

Movement:
☑ Slowly lower your body until your upper arm is parallel to the floor.
☑ Contracting the triceps muscles, slowly return to the starting position stopping just short of the arms fully extending.

Key Points:
☑ Slowly lower your body until your upper arm is parallel to the floor.
☑ Contracting the triceps muscles, slowly return to the starting position stopping just short of the arms fully extending.

Dumbbell Double Biceps Curl

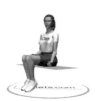

Starting Position:
☑ Sit on a bench/chair with both feet in front of your body and your back straight.
☑ Hold a dumbbell in each hand with your arms at each side and palms facing forward.

Movement:
☑ While contracting the biceps muscles, raise the weights toward your shoulders, stopping just short of the weights touching the shoulders.
☑ Slowly return to the starting position.

Key Points:
☑ Exhale while lifting the weights.
☑ Inhale when returning to the starting position.
☑ Your upper arms should remain stationary throughout the exercise.
☑ Perform 12 to 15 repetitions and immediately go to the next exercise.

Dumbbell Behind-The-Head Triceps Extension

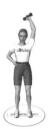

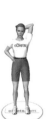

Starting Position:
☑ Stand with a dumbbell in your right hand with your left hand on your hip.
☑ Press the weight over your head until your right arm is almost straight with a slight bend in the elbow at the top position.
☑ Do not allow the weight to touch your head or neck.

Movement:
☑ Slowly bend your elbow, lowering the weight until your arm forms a 90-degree angle behind your head, stopping before the weight touches your back.
☑ While contracting the triceps muscles, slowly return to the starting position.

Key Points:
☑ Exhale while returning to the starting position.
☑ Inhale when lowering the weight.
☑ After completing the set on the right side, repeat on the left side.
☑ This exercise is not to be performed with very heavy dumbbells. The technique is more important than the weight.

SLEEK AND SEXY SHOULDERS

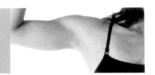

Machine Lateral Raise

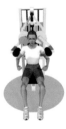

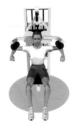

Starting Position:
☑ Adjust yourself in the machine as per the instructions.

Movement:
☑ Contracting the shoulder muscles, extend the arms out to the side, stopping when your upper arm is parallel with the floor.
☑ Slowly return to the starting position, stopping just short of the weight stack touching.

Key Points:
☑ Exhale while lifting the weight.
☑ Inhale while returning to the starting position.
☑ Try to maintain a neutral spine throughout the entire range of motion and keep the shoulder blades squeezed together.
☑ Do not round the upper back or let the chest cave in.

Fitball Dumbbell Shoulder Press

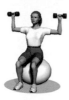

Starting Position:
☑ While holding dumbbells or cans, sit on the ball or on a chair or bench, with feet flat on the floor.
☑ The upper arm should be parallel with the floor with a 90-degree angle at the elbows.

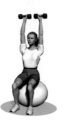

Movement:
☑ While contracting the shoulder muscles, raise the weights toward the ceiling, stopping when the arms are fully extended, with a slight bend in the elbows.
☑ Slowly return to the starting position.

Key Points:
☑ Exhale while lifting the weights.
☑ Inhale when returning to the starting position.
☑ Perform 12 to 15 repetitions and immediately go on to the next exercise.

Dumbbell Bent-Over Rear Delt Raise

Starting Position:
☑ Sit on a bench or chair and bend forward to a 45-degree angle.
☑ Hold a dumbbell or can in each hand with your arms hanging at your sides and the palms facing one another.
☑ Pull your shoulders back and lift your chest up.

Movement:
☑ While contracting the rear shoulder muscles, lift your arms out to the sides until they are at shoulder height.
☑ Slowly return to the starting position, stopping just short of your arms touching your legs.

Key Points:
☑ Exhale while lifting the weights.
☑ Inhale when returning to the starting position.
☑ If your arms gravitate forward or backward, you will not be isolating the rear shoulder muscles.
☑ Do not round your upper back or shoulders.
☑ Do not allow your chest to cave in.
☑ If you're a beginner, perform each movement slowly and at your own pace.
☑ Try for 10 to 12 repetitions on each movement and take your time moving from one exercise to the next.
☑ Perform only two sets of each movement on two alternate days per week.

Motivation
SOLUTIONS

When you start on your weight management journey, choose a route that is filled with supportive people, resources and tools, and you can succeed.

Weight Loss
Begins with You

☑ **Visualize success.** Dieting isn't easy, but setting goals and staying committed can change your life. Dream of the life you want and visualize what it will look like – what you will be doing, how you will look and how you will be living. Find a picture that best illustrates what that life will be like and place it in a conspicuous place.

☑ **Find your passion.** Love the journey. Do everything that brings you closer to your goals with passion. Write down three reasons why you are passionate about getting healthier. Start your journey with determination. Take small steps to start. And don't let anyone distract you from being the best you can be.

☑ **Educate yourself.** Read articles, books and any other motivational material that interests you and can help you be more informed. Arm yourself with the tools that you need to help you on the journey.

☑ **Get support from others.** Whether it's family, friends or coworkers – surround yourself with supportive people who encourage you along the way. Find private, anonymous support online in the form of message boards or support groups. Share your successes and challenges and be inspired by others who are on the same journey as you. Join in as often as you need to keep motivated … and make some friends in the process.

☑ **Start with small changes.** The small stuff can add up to big results. At lunch, order your chicken sandwich or hamburger without mayonnaise, or decide not to eat carbs after 7 p.m. Commit to taking a 10-minute walk each day and increase your time each week. Gradual changes help you feel better about yourself as you embark on the journey to reach your goals.

☑ **Move beyond a "bad" day.** Everyone has moments of weakness. If you have a "bad" day, accept it as one bad moment and move on to your next great moment.

☑ **Reward yourself.** When you incorporate a healthy habit or reach a milestone, reward yourself with a non-food prize, such as a manicure, bubble bath or sleeping in. Treat yourself to anything you enjoy for making it one step closer to your goal.

☑ **Know that you're worth it!** "Fat" is not a personality trait. Write down 10 positive adjectives that describe you and read them aloud each day. Find a quote that inspires you and read it to yourself often. Do whatever it takes to keep your inner voice positive.

Real People, Real Results.

Challenge:	Start Weight: 148 lbs
Overcoming a high-stress life	End Weight: 126 lbs.
	Pounds Lost: 22

Results not typical.

Keli Lost 22 lbs. on the GI Diet

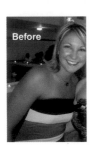

Keli R. was living life in the fast lane until an unexpected turn of events slowed her down.

"My dad got sick one day, went to the emergency room and had double-bypass heart surgery the next day," she says. "Living a high-stress life, being on the road all the time and eating fast food at every meal nearly did him in, but luckily he was able to fully recover."

While watching her dad undergo major surgery, the former all-state volleyball champion vowed to improve her own health.

"I realized I needed to step up my game and get serious about losing weight, getting in shape and making sure that what I put into my body was really helping it."

Keli found that the eDiets Glycemic Impact plan best matched her lifestyle. The 21-year-old student from Texas, loved that she could access eDiets.com whenever and wherever she wanted and take advantage of the customizable tools, meal plans and support boards.

"The customizable shopping lists, the support groups, the multiple creative and exciting meals – it was something that I couldn't pass up and that I knew would keep me on track. I love the online meetings. It's great to have expert advice right at your disposal."

On the GI Diet, Keli was eating five to six times a day and enjoying an array of different delicious choices. From the moment she woke up until she went to sleep, she felt satisfied.

"Who could pass up a diet that lets you eat all the time? The food choices are great; preparation is easy; and the GI Diet has been a great way for me to get back on track with healthy eating and feeling better about myself."

Although Keli had been an avid volleyball player for most of her life, she gradually became less active because of her hectic schedule. Once she got her diet on track, her energy level went up, and she felt like exercising again.

"I love doing cardio now, and it has made such a huge difference. I've started doing yoga and Pilates," she says. "And I've loved the way that it's started to streamline my body. Working out makes me feel fabulous – it's become a relaxing thing for me."

		Start Weight: 145 lbs.
	**Challenge:** Finding support	End Weight: 112 lbs. Pounds Lost: 33

Results not typical.

From Flab to Fab, She's 33 lbs. Lighter!

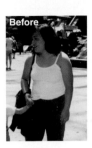
Before

These before and after photos tell a tale of two Dianes.

There's the drab Diane T. who went out of her way to avoid mirrors. When she walked down the street, she kept her head down. At 5 feet tall, she found herself depressed, even inconsolable, when she reached 157 pounds.

Now Diane is smiling again. Though it took her 10 years to pack on those pounds, she was able to work them off in six short months. The new Diane is spunky, sexy and full of confidence. She's transformed herself from a flabby 145 pounds to a sleek and slender 112.

"Everyone is asking me how I did it," the curvy Californian says. "It's a wonderful feeling. I'm more confident and feeling more comfortable in my skin than I ever have. I'm at a weight I haven't been in over 11 years."

It wasn't the first time Diane called upon eDiets for help with her weight woes. She first reached out to the online weight-loss program back in 2000. Although she had everything she needed to succeed, the 27-year-old secretary admits she failed to attain the kind of results she achieved the second time around.

The reason her earlier efforts bottomed out? Diane says it's because she didn't use the always-active eDiets support boards. With more than 100 boards spanning a wealth of topics and lifestyles, there's something for everyone. Diane never thought she'd benefit much from posting messages on the eDiets' online boards, but it proved to be the resource that finally helped her unload the extra baggage.

"It's the emotional support and motivation I got from others that drove me to continue. Having people there who know how you feel, who keep on pushing you to better yourself is amazing. There's nothing like it."

Despite her distaste for exercise, Diane joined a gym. At first, the weight room and machines intimidated her, but that's all changed. She is now an exercise enthusiast.

"When I have a bad day, I go work out, and it relieves stress and tension."

While she keeps a balanced regimen, Diane says her heart is in weight lifting, partly because it hastens physical changes. Diane insists that if she can do it, you can do it — it's simply a matter of wanting it badly enough. "How bad do you want it?" she asks.

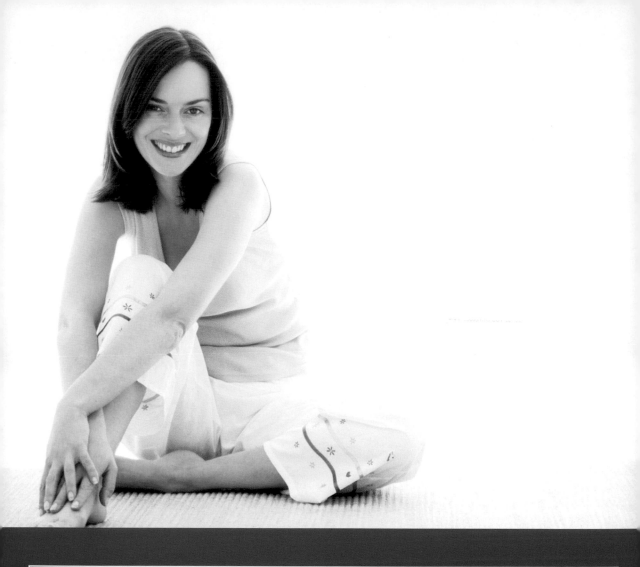

Find Your
Motivation

You've got to start somewhere. The stories
and tools on the following pages will show you
exactly where you need to be.

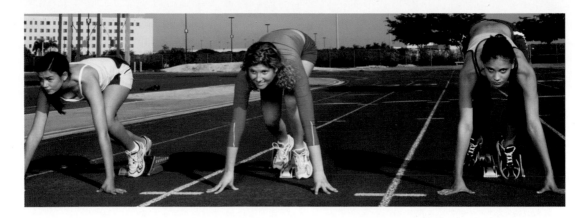

The dictionary lists "that which gives purpose and direction to behavior" and "drive or incentive" as definitions of motivation. What drives you and gives you purpose? Find your source of motivation by answering that question, and remember the incentive as you embark on your weight-management journey.

Take action by starting with these strategies:

☑ **Put it in writing.** A good way to increase your chances of following through on your intentions is to put your plans in writing. Make a contract with yourself. Identify specific goals — write down how much weight you want to lose, how you plan to accomplish your goals and when you plan to start. Now sign on the dotted line and keep the contract where you can't help but see it every day, like on the fridge or taped to your mirror.

☑ **Let yourself love healthy food.** Eating healthy food doesn't have to be boring or bland. Sure, there are people who eat bean sprouts, cottage cheese, tofu and raw vegetables, but that doesn't have to become your eating style. Some people follow a specific diet plan, and others opt to omit certain types of foods or cooking styles. For example, simply giving up fried foods can be a real asset to your weight-loss efforts. Remember, your diet doesn't have to be extreme to get results.

☑ **If not for yourself...** Family, friends and loved ones are great motivators for staying on track. You need to self-motivate, but "doing it for them" can keep you focused on losing weight. Imagine how much more energy you'll have to give to your children, for example. Or how much longer of a romantic walk you'll be able to go on next time you're at the beach with your partner.

Simply giving up fried foods can be a real asset to your weight-loss efforts.

☑ **Mix it up.** Are your favorite healthful foods out of season or simply unavailable in your part of the country? It can be hard to find good, flavorful fruit during the winter. Order a box of oranges or grapefruits from sunny Florida. Or purchase frozen blueberries and strawberries to toss into salads or on cereal. Getting food in the mail can be fun, and adding new flavors to your diet while still maintaining a healthy eating plan just makes it all the more fun and easy to follow.

☑ **Fun workouts?** Yes. The best way to boost your exercise motivation is to make exercising an activity you actually enjoy doing. Scan the workout videos or check out your gym's class schedule until you find something that sounds like fun, such as boxing or Tai Chi. Keep trying new activities until you find one that really has you looking forward to breaking a sweat. Think back to your favorite sports in school: Did volleyball challenge you? Perhaps it was tennis' one-on-one attitude that you liked. Get out there and play a sport if you don't want to join a gym, work out at home with a video, or just jog or walk in your neighborhood.

☑ **Find safety in numbers.** Sometimes having someone to share the experience with you is all you need to stay on track. If your spouse, sibling or friend also wants to lose weight, consider working toward your goals together. Many times it helps to have a co-worker who is also determined to get healthier. You can start on the same day and support each other when the going gets tough. The added responsibility of meeting someone for a workout every day or reporting your meals to that person can be a terrific way to stick to your plan.

☑ **Weigh your options.** Make a list of all the reasons losing weight is important to you (e.g., looking great, feeling better about yourself, reducing your risk for disease, having more energy — whatever motivates you). Just thinking about all the amazing things you'll be doing for yourself can motivate you.

☑ **Listen up.** Pay attention to the response you get from people around you. As you begin to lose weight, the compliments you get from friends (even strangers) — and the differences you notice in yourself — will keep you motivated for the duration.

☑ **Consider the fringe benefits.** You already know about those health and fitness benefits, but how about better sex? A study at Duke University found that moderate weight loss in men (8 to 20 pounds) resulted in significant improvements in "sexual functioning and satisfaction." Research has also shown that regular exercisers have higher levels of desire and an enhanced ability to be aroused and achieve orgasm. Exercise improves blood flow throughout the body, and increased circulation is related to heightened sexual desire in both men and women.

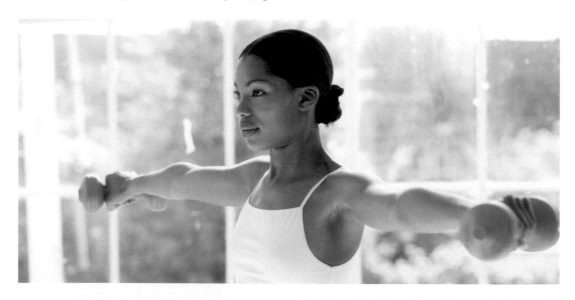

Turning Dieting Mistakes
into Motivators

Those who succeed in losing weight and making the change to a healthy lifestyle are those who handle mistakes the best. Seize the opportunity to focus on the positive – turn every diet "mistake" into an action item that guides and motivates you. Choose a few from the list below to get you started and prevent mistakes before they happen.

1 Choose a diet that you can adhere to for the rest of your life.

2 Eat in moderation and avoid counting calories.

3 Limit yourself to eating out only once a week.

4 Drink plenty of water.

5 Eliminate sugary drinks, such as lemonade, soft drinks, gourmet coffees and fruity drinks.

6 Eat less bread, pasta and potatoes and enjoy more fruits and vegetables.

7 Consume more fresh foods than processed foods.

8 Don't overcook vegetables – preserve their vitamins.

9 Have a positive attitude.

10 Have a plan.

11 Be aware of the nutritional benefits of what you consume.

12 Stop eating when you are full.

13 Eat reasonable portions on your plate, and don't go back for seconds.

14 Enjoy breakfast; don't skip it.

15 Eat the right portions, stay satisfied and still lose weight!

16 Don't let a "bad" day derail your success.

17 Believe you have the ability to change.

18 Know that you are beautiful.

19 Finish tasks you start – you are successful in so many facets of your life.

20 Live each day to the fullest "now " and "when you are thinner."

21 Think of exercise as a fun and energizing activity, not a "must-do" or chore.

22 Be a participant in sports, as well as an observer.

23 Watch less TV.

24 Buy healthy snacks for the kids and yourself.

25 Have vegetables and/or fruit with each meal.

26 Think of the way you eat as a lifestyle change, not a "diet."

27 Visualize yourself living a healthy lifestyle.

28 Take a multivitamin and proper supplements.

29 Never give up.

30 Don't wait for tomorrow. Start now!

Push Through a
Plateau

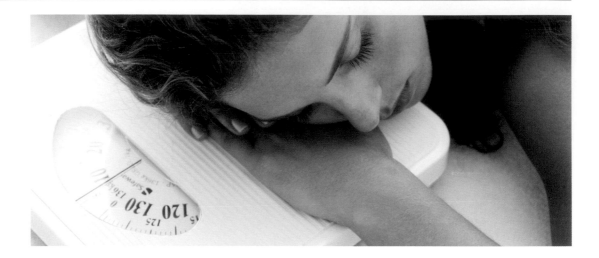

There will come a time when your body readjusts to the number of calories you are consuming and becomes more accustomed to your regular exercise regimen. When your weight loss bottoms out, you may panic that you have worked so hard and now won't be able to lose any more weight. Rest assured; there are many things you can do to get off that weight-loss plateau.

▷ Consume Calories

Consuming too few calories causes your body to go into starvation mode, and as a result, your body holds on tightly to all of the calories it can, thinking that it is protecting you from starvation. Listen to your body. This is a natural mechanism. You may need to add more calories to your diet in order to lose weight safely and steadily.

▷ Keep a Food Diary

A great way to figure out what is actually going on is to track your food intake. You automatically become more conscious of what you are eating when you know that you need to record it, and when you review, you can identify patterns. For example, you may see that you are eating more calories than you ever realized during your work day (picking up candy at your co-worker's desk, having a piece of your boss's birthday cake, and sneaking a few of the potato chips your office mate offered to you). Another pattern may be that on the days when you skip breakfast, you consume more calories in the afternoon than on the days when you eat breakfast. It is important to identify your own eating patterns, habits and triggers for overeating. A food diary is the perfect tool to help you.

▷ Change Your Eating Patterns

You have kept your food diary, you're convinced that your calorie consumption is in your target range, you're still following your plan, and you're sticking to a strict exercise regimen – what now? The answer is change.

Try switching your meals around. Eat what's scheduled for breakfast at lunchtime, and vice versa. Or try breakfast for dinner. This will undoubtedly help you cut some additional calories, which will help you lose weight.

▷ Vary Your Workouts

Walking four times a week is great, but your body may have become accustomed to that routine. First, try to increase either the walking speed or the distance. Or, instead of just walking, try alternating five minutes of walking with five minutes of jogging. Maybe ride a bike a couple of days each week. Try a new class at the gym or a new machine to vary your cardiovascular workout. If you normally use the treadmill, give the elliptical trainer a try.

Weight-bearing activities are extremely important and can help speed up your metabolism. Muscle burns more calories than fat. Therefore, the more lean body mass you have, the more calories you burn, even when you're not working out. If you aren't doing any strength training, start slowly. You can start by using your own body weight as resistance, using elastic bands, or by purchasing light hand weights.

▷ Stay Motivated

Stay motivated. Are you feeling better? Do your clothes fit better? While your scale may not register a weight loss, you may be losing inches. Judge weight loss by clothing fit and inches lost, not just the scale. Keep in mind that you have already been successful! Think about the pounds that you have lost so far and the new healthy behaviors you are now following. Keep your chin up, visualize yourself at your goal weight and you will succeed!

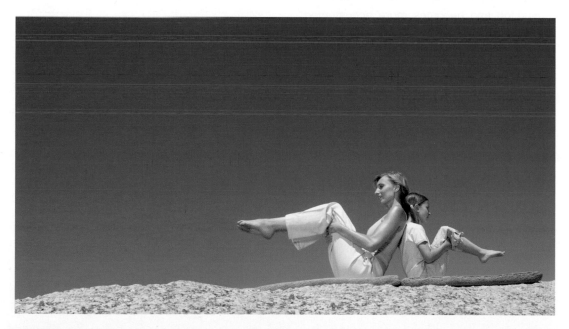

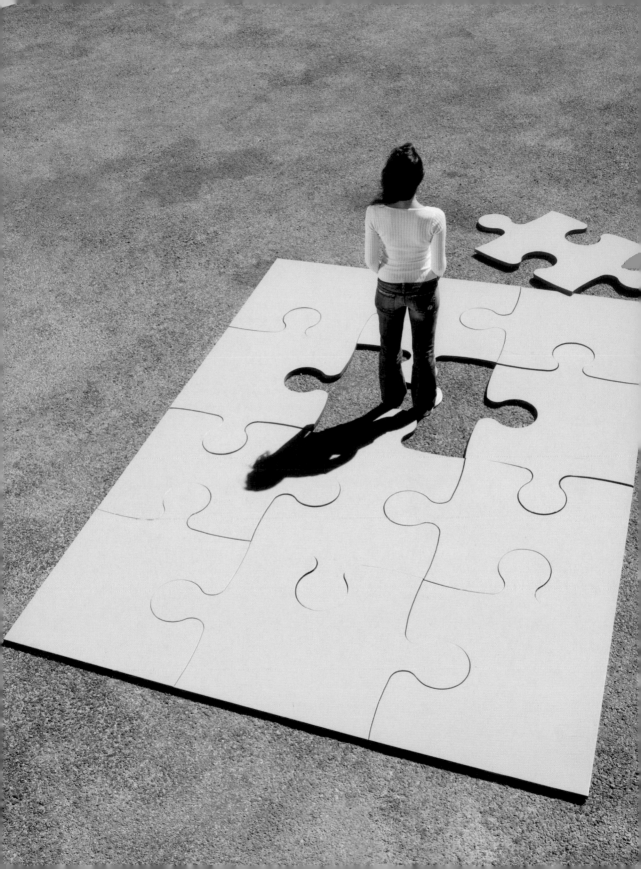

Be Prepared for
Temptation

Foods that don't fit into your healthy lifestyle are everywhere, but you can resist when you're confronted with temptation.

Family functions, the "goody" table at work and the candy at the supermarket checkout are just a few places where your resolve is tested. Dealing with these "tests" takes practice and patience, but when you stand up for your needs instead of buckling under pressure, you'll gain a sense of pride and stay on your path to weight loss.

When temptation arises, just say, "No, thank you."

You can increase your chances of sticking to your guns when confronted with food temptations.

There are three magic words that can empower you when temptation arises – just say, "No, thank you." Say those words nicely and firmly when others pressure you to eat something that's not on your plan. You don't have to make excuses or feel guilty. Just remember the power of your pound-shedding principles. And when your friends and family understand how important a healthy lifestyle is to you, they'll come around.

Our friends, relatives and coworkers influence us in many ways, from how we dress to what we watch on TV. But when it comes to eating healthfully and losing weight, it's all about you. Whatever your reason for pursuing weight-loss – improving your self-image, fitting into a special outfit or just getting healthier – visualize those goals when faced with temptation and remind your loved ones.

A great way to ward off temptation is to be armed at all times with healthy snacks that fit your plan. Toss a few pieces of fruit, crunchy vegetables, granola bars or some low-fat yogurt in a cooler and stash it in the car. You'll be less likely to stop at the drive-thru when you're stuck in traffic and hunger strikes.

Keeping your eyes on the prize is a super way to resist temptation. Chocolate cake sure looks delicious, but you'll look even better when you're healthier and fitter. Visualize yourself in the way you want to look and remind yourself of that image when the going gets tough. Make an inspirational quote your mantra and say it to yourself when you need motivation.

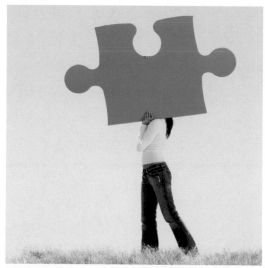

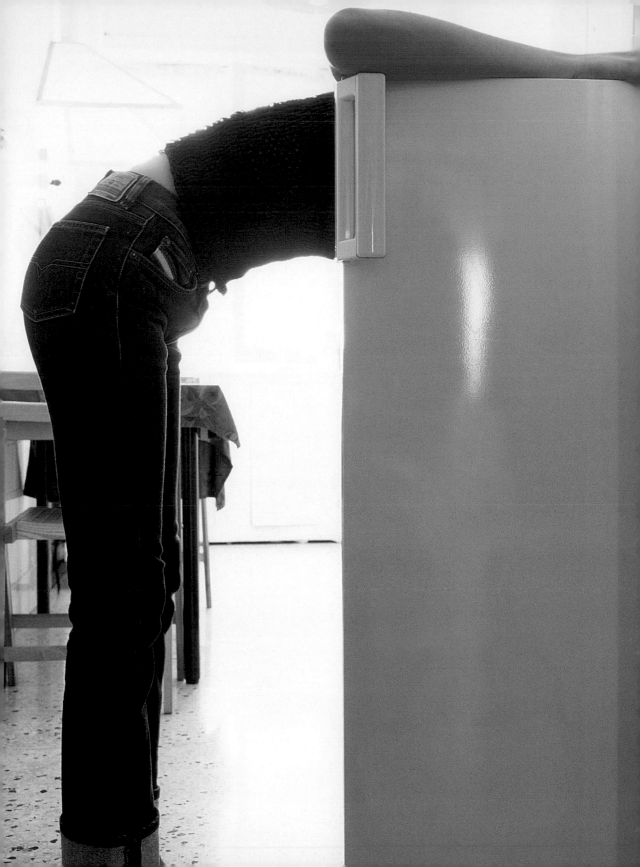

Willpower:
Find It. Use It.

What is willpower and where can you find it? Before we answer those questions, let's start with a definiton of "willpower." The American Heritage Dictionary defines willpower as: "The strength of will to carry out one's decisions, wishes or plans." That makes it a bit clearer, but what exactly is "will?" It is defined as: "The mental faculty by which one deliberately chooses or decides upon a course of action. Diligent purposefulness, determination, self-control and self-discipline."

After a closer examination of what the words really mean, we can see that most of us are never really without willpower. If you are a living, functioning human being – aware enough to want to go on a diet – then you possess the "mental faculty by which you deliberately choose." The choices you make are a direct result of your willpower.

The definition of willpower is purposeful determination. Finding your purpose is another essential aspect of a weight-loss effort.

How many times has a diet failed you? Most of us feel the need to make excuses when we don't see the results that we desire, and "having no willpower" is where most dieters place blame. Help your diet work for you by exploring the concept of willpower. Find out how to get it and how to keep it working for you.

You must know WHY you are doing this, what you want to get out of it and how it is going to impact your life and the lives of others. Knowing your purpose is vital to this journey's success. Once you have found your purpose, you must be determined to realize it.

▷ You Already Have It!

Now that you know what willpower is, you still need to know where to find it. Willpower lies within. Defining your purpose and believing that you have the determination to realize it opens up vast inner stores of willpower. You have it inside you; you only need to reach in there and harness it.

Now that you know what it is and where to find it, learn how to keep it and make it work for you. There are tools you can use to help you make the most of the willpower you have. Try a mantra: "I have WILLpower." Begin every day by saying this to yourself. Say it as you look in the mirror and while you are getting ready for work in the morning.

▷ Know That You Can

Self-discovery is the key to long-term weight loss. You need to discover the real sources of the energies that drive you toward food. When you identify these sources, you can create a plan for handling, managing, healing and transforming them. Once you do, they will not generate the energies that drive you to overeat.

When you are faced with food challenges, remind yourself that you are fueled by "WILLpower," and that you don't need whatever treat is tempting you. Know that you can, believe that you WILL and DO what you are determined to do.

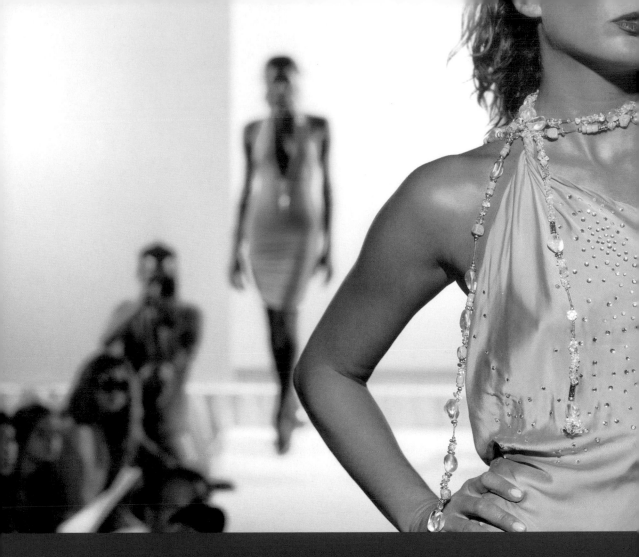

Feeling **Good**

Whether you need to lose 10 pounds or 100, you should be armed with proper motivational tools.

Don't Run Out of
Self-Esteem

Self-esteem is an attitude of acceptance and non-judgment toward yourself and others. Self-esteem is essential for psychological survival. It is the ability to form an identity and then attach a value to it. You have the capacity to define who you are and then make a decision as to whether or not you like that identity.

Our self-esteem may have been shaped by our parents early in life. However, it is later in life when we have the ability to re-condition the things we have learned, if we so desire. As adults, we can no longer blame our parents for their mistakes. As adults, we have choices. We either live as victims, or we do something to better today and our future.

Begin taking note of your reaction to the situations in which you find yourself. Focus on the type of thinking you are engaged in and how it relates to your feelings about the situation. Make an attempt to alter your thinking about each situation, and then become aware of the change in the related emotion.

For example, after eating a couple of cookies, rather than allowing yourself to have negative thoughts and then eating the rest of the box, tell yourself, "I only had two cookies, and it's better than eating the entire box." Think about the consequences of the first scenario. This type of thinking will cause great damage to your sense of self-esteem and self-worth.

Changing the way you think will have a profound effect on your overall well-being. Flexible thinking and self-praise are the keys to a positive sense of self-worth. It is important to begin using positive statements to enhance your self-esteem. Learning to think in a positive manner takes practice. It will not happen overnight, but anything worthwhile takes time and patience.

It feels so much better to look in the mirror and say, "I am beautiful" instead of allowing negative thoughts that diminish your self-esteem. The manner in which you interpret your life has an enormous effect on your self-esteem. Start improving it today!

MOTIVATIONAL STATEMENTS

Use positive statements to help enhance your self-esteem.

☑ Appreciate the **natural blessings** with which you were born.

☑ Find the **goodness in yourself** and de-emphasize flaws that cannot be changed.

☑ Concentrate on **good health** rather than on pleasing anyone other than yourself.

☑ Know that the outer layer is only skin deep; it's **what's inside** that counts.

☑ Behave in a way that's consistent with **your own values**, not those of others.

☑ Learn to appreciate your own **uniqueness**.

☑ The grass is never really greener on the other side of the fence; it just depends on how much **nurturing the gardener** gives it.

☑ **Take time** to smell the roses.

Get Your Eating
On Track!

Introducing Nutrition Tracker℠ from eDiets.com®
It's quick. It's easy. And it's absolutely __FREE!__

This handy nutrition tracking tool makes it easy to track what you eat. Just enter the foods you eat each day and Nutrition Tracker does the rest. It counts daily calories, carbs, sugars, proteins, fats and more.

As you continue to use Nutrition Tracker, it develops a profile of your eating habits that will tell you what you've been doing right … and what you could be doing better.

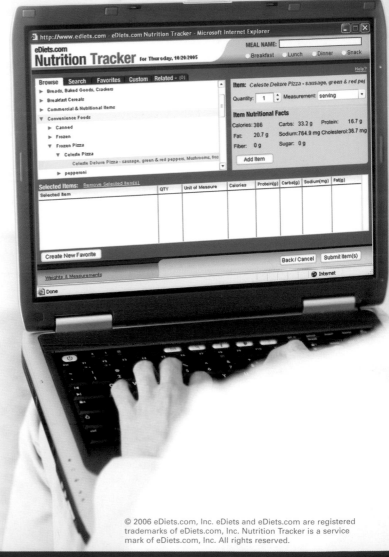

© 2006 eDiets.com, Inc. eDiets and eDiets.com are registered trademarks of eDiets.com, Inc. Nutrition Tracker is a service mark of eDiets.com, Inc. All rights reserved.

Get your diet back on track. Try Nutrition Tracker today!
FREE from eDiets.com.

Challenge: Increasing low energy levels	Start Weight: 207 lbs. End Weight: 155 lbs. Pounds Lost: 52

Results not typical.

From Frumpy to Fabulous

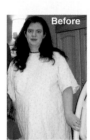

Amy N. believes it's what's on the inside that counts, but she didn't let that philosophy stop her from renovating the outside by dropping a whopping 52 pounds.

Even when she hit her highest weight of 247 pounds during pregnancy, the 28-year-old managed to make the best of things. Although she sometimes ran out of energy, she wasn't completely miserable. She had two children and a caring husband who loved her through thick and thin. She could have stayed overweight and been happy, but she didn't want to run the risk of developing obesity-related illnesses such as heart disease, diabetes and more.

"I'm not really a fan of the idea that fat makes you unhappy," Amy says. "I certainly had less energy and wasn't always very confident about how I looked. But I personally feel it's what's on the inside that counts. I was hoping to make those match."

And that's just what the Colorado audiologist did with the help of eDiets. The online weight-loss program gave her a personalized meal plan that provided customized shopping lists, recipes and menus, along with 24/7 peer and professional support. Within months, Amy's weight went from 207 to 155 pounds.

By unloading 52 pounds from her 5-foot, 10-inch figure and dropping from a size 18/20 to a size 10, our super slimmer feels better than ever.

"It helped to have the structure that the eDiets program provided. I probably could've come up with something of my own, but I don't think it would have been as effective. It would have been easier for me to cheat on myself for one thing. It's also nice to be able to go online and plug my weight in every week and see the graphs and steps going down, seeing my success that way."

As for working out, she went to a water aerobics class. Because most of the people were overweight, Amy didn't feel self-conscious in a bathing suit. She enjoys hiking and walking around a lake close to her home and chasing around her two small children.

Her husband, David, was also a big part of her success, she said. He was supportive, congratulating her on even the smallest losses. It was the praise and the progress that kept her on board for the long haul.

Unleash Your
Mind's Power

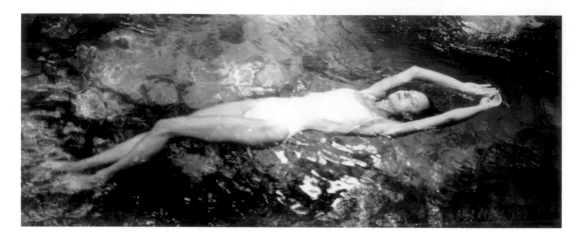

Imagery is the ancient art of using words and sounds to take you on an imaginary journey. It creates a state of mind and body that provides great emotional and physical benefits. The sick and injured use imagery to enhance healing. Top athletes use it in their pursuit of peak performance. Everyday people who want to be more effective, optimize their potential for success and learn how to win at life can try imagery. Imagery is said to be the primary language of the unconscious mind.

▷ The Ultimate Tool

Imagery is a tool that can change your life. Nothing is safer and more powerful than change powered by strategic mental imagery.

Imagery exercises can recharge your emotional batteries, help you connect with your inner power and teach you how to mobilize your own resources. They can help you change the way you live your life forever — from the inside-out.

"Whatever you give your attention to grows." That old saying is true, whether you are talking about your garden, children, ideas, hopes or fears. Imagery allows you to focus your attention on your strengths and explore your potential. After all, you are so much more potential than you are reality. But we tend to draw our own boundaries regarding what we do and what we think. Imagery activities serve as a rehearsal for real-life experiences.

You will never be who you want to be by remaining who you are.

Regarding weight control, you can use imagery as a powerful tool for change. Use it to help you learn, to control those forces within you that influence daily eating and health decisions. Imagery can encourage healthy decision-making by increasing your sense of confidence and allowing you to experience more power and control.

Because we are all creatures of habit, the most difficult first step toward change involves trying new thoughts and behaviors. Imagery does this very well. For many, an introduction to new thoughts and behaviors turns into a lifelong relationship with change.

▷ Who Do You Want to Be?

You will never be who you want to be by remaining who you are. If you want to get healthy and reclaim your body, then you must change. And imagery is a powerful and effective agent for change. It is not an attempt to create something that isn't there. Imagery is a way to strengthen what already exists.

A growing body of medical research continues to demonstrate the power of imagery. Dr. Andrew Weil, one of today's top wellness doctors, is a passionate advocate of imagery. He and others have found imagery to be a powerful influence on every major control system in the body.

Imagery can help change your life forever – from the inside-out.

"Imagery can be a helpful tool in up to 90 percent of all problems people bring to their doctors, from headaches, back pain and allergies to serious, life-threatening illnesses like cancer and obesity," Dr. Weil says. "It doesn't replace good medical care, but it can definitely make good medical care more effective."

Dr. Weil says, "To the extent that mind-body therapies can reduce stress and promote positive attitudes, they can ease symptoms and improve the quality of life for people suffering from many different conditions."

▷ The Right Brain

A powerful tool for self-awareness and change, imagery lets you play an important role in your own mind. It uses the symbolic language of the right brain, allowing you to communicate with your unconscious mind. It can make you deeply aware of how your thoughts, feelings and habits influence your choices, body and health.

You already have the power to change. All you have to do is tap your inner resources by focusing your attention in the right direction. Imagery is an excellent way to make that happen. Imagine that!

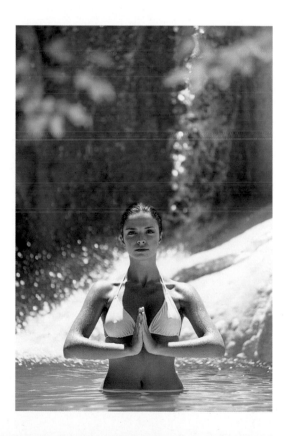

You Can't Do It
Without You

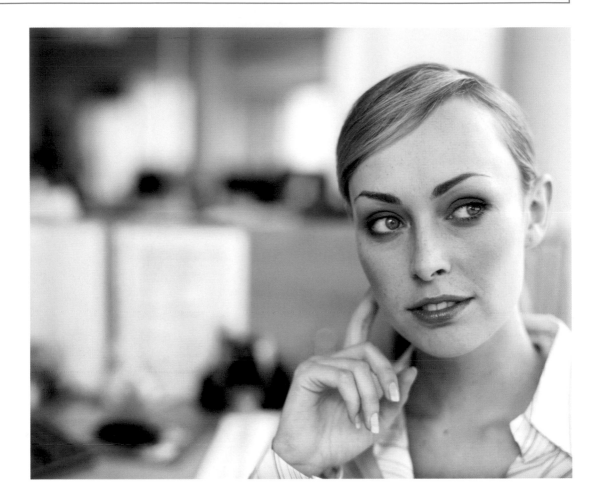

Question: What is the single most important tool for successful weight loss?

If your answer was a good diet, an effective exercise program, counting calories or even a support group, you would have named some very useful tools. However, there's more to it than those tools.

What is this elusive but crucial weight-loss tool? YOU. To be more specific, knowledge about yourself is the factor that is most often left out of diet programs.

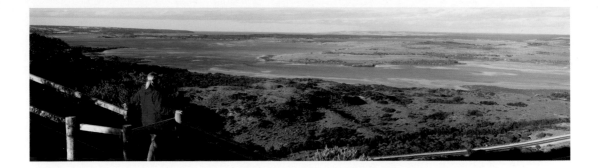

Centuries ago, a wise Chinese teacher named Lao-Tzu said it this way: "He who knows others is wise; he who knows himself is enlightened." You may know a lot about exercise and diet and follow a detailed weight-loss program, but knowing what makes you tick (your needs, inner hungers, addictions, fears, hopes and ultimately what makes you eat uncontrollably) goes a long way in achieving long-term weight loss.

"He who knows others is wise; he who knows himself is enlightened."

Imagine that you want to go from New York to California because a billion-dollar inheritance is waiting for you. The only way to travel is by car, and you do not know how to drive. Then someone gives you a new car. What would you do? Wouldn't you take some serious driving lessons immediately and learn as much as you could about driving and basic car maintenance?

Well, weight loss is far more complex than driving across the country, but most dieters know far less about themselves than they do about their own cars.

▷ Explore Your Inner Self

You are a complex and wonderful being. You have needs and wants, fears and hopes, desires and expectations that all have a direct effect on what and how you eat. Did you know that a little self-exploration could make a giant difference in your ability to change your eating habits?

A big weight-loss tip: If you are stuck on the way to your weight goal, then self-knowledge is probably what you need to have a breakthrough. How do you get this knowledge? Try answering the questions below. They will move you in the right direction.

Weight-Related Self-Knowledge Questions

The more you know about yourself, the more weight you can lose.

- What is my greatest **inner hunger**, other than food?
- What childhood trauma still affects my emotions, eating habits and **self-image**?
- What major **life risk** have I been unwilling to take?
- What **intense feelings** most influence my overeating?
- What am I willing to do to learn about and **productively manage** those feelings?
- To what degree do I still **fear growing** up?
- How often do I blame others for my current **life situation** instead of taking responsibility for my choices?
- How does my weight **help me hide** from life?

Dress Slimmer, **Look Thinner**

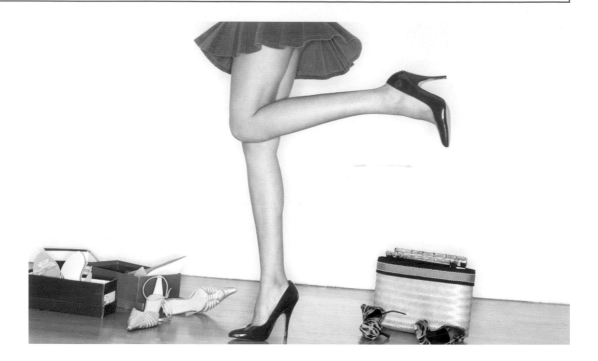

Introducing the secret ingredient in low-fat dressing: It's called fashion. That's right, fashion, and it's time to pour it all out and reveal how it can work for you.

As you progress toward your healthy weight goal, imagine for a moment if every time you slipped into an outfit you automatically looked younger and thinner. Chances are your closet would become your new best friend. When it comes to looking slimmer, sexy and better than ever, you don't have to look further than your wardrobe.

The power of fashion is often overlooked. How you look to others entirely depends on what you wear and how you wear it. Having good manners and a pleasing appearance are the most important characteristics you can possess in making good impressions. Most people unknowingly add to their weight every time they get dressed. Instead of magnifying negative features, it's easy to accentuate the positive. What do you see when you look in the mirror? Are your clothes helping you look your best, or are you adding the illusion of extra pounds?

People come in all shapes and sizes. A style of clothes that flatters one body type may be wrong for another. Tall, short, big, small, narrow or wide, there are tricks to

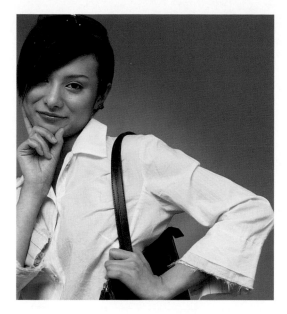

transforming your clothes to flatter your figure.

The single most important piece in the fashion game, however, is having confidence. When you are self-assured and comfortable in your clothes, it shows. Fashion trends are started by people who are sure of themselves. They feel good, and, in return, look good in their clothes. There is nothing more pleasing to the eye then a person who walks around with her head held high. Feel free to experiment and use your sense of style to your advantage.

Here are some basic fashion tactics you can use to look better and boost your confidence and body image.

☑ **Long silhouettes.** Whether it be long pants or skirts, a longer hemline will always lengthen and slim the body. Look for a straight or boot-cut styles when choosing slacks or jeans; they create a smoother line. Tapered cuts or pants that cut close to the ankles will actually make you look bigger around the waist and hip area and create an exaggerated V-shape, which is opposite of what you're trying to achieve.

If you choose a pant leg that is fuller at the knees and widens slightly at the calves and ankles, you're creating a more proportional shape, which is extremely flattering on any size. The shoe you wear is also important in elongating the frame.

☑ **Wear solid fabrics.** Wearing one color from head to toe is more slimming than combining solids and patterns.

☑ **Stick to dark colors.** Darker, richer colors are generally more slimming than lighter neutrals. Compare different shades and see what best complements your skin. Wearing colors like brown, navy, gray or plum not only makes you look slimmer, but it's also a quick and easy way to look chic and sophisticated.

☑ **Wear high heels.** The higher, the better. Heels will help you appear taller and thinner because they slim the silhouette. If you don't like high heels, then choose a low-heeled shoe that is cut low on the instep.

☑ **Accessorize.** Wearing a scarf, necklace, earrings or choker takes the concentration off the body. Plus sizes look great in bold, chunky

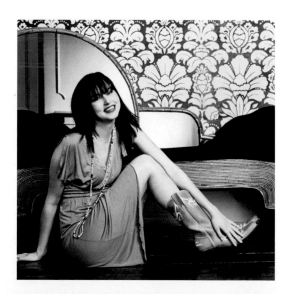

jewelry, so if your personal style ranges from eccentric to ethnic to artistic, go for those one-of-a-kind pieces, but keep proportion in mind.

☑ **Choose V-necklines.** They make you look leaner and longer. V-necks and low necklines show off the clavicle, or collarbone, and help create a slimming effect.

☑ **Wear clothes that accentuate the positive.** Just because you've got curves doesn't mean you have to hide them. If you've got a round backside, show it off in a great pencil skirt. If you've got great cleavage, flaunt it in a low-cut button-down shirt.

☑ **Always look neat and clean.** Keep your nails clean and evenly trimmed, take care of your clothes, de-fuzz your sweaters, buy a good deodorant and make sure your shoes are polished and unscuffed.

☑ **Wear colors that work for you.** Experiment with different colors and stick with palettes that look best on you. If you're into all black, use feminine, colorful accessories to offset the darkness.

☑ **Wear clothes that fit.** Maximize your figure with pants that fit smoothly and are the right length; wear shirts that don't gape at the buttons; and wear sweaters that aren't too big. Shop for the perfect fit or have them tailored to fit.

☑ **Wear the right makeup.** A good rule of thumb is light for the day, heavier for evening and sheer for sports.

☑ **Rely on your own style.** Every woman has to cultivate her own, personal style. Add only a few trendy pieces to outfits that define your style.

☑ **Plan before you buy.** Buying odds and ends on sale may seem to save you money, but it will leave you searching for clothes. Buy entire outfits instead of only separates.

☑ **Keep it under wraps.** Buy slips that fit, make sure your bra fits properly and that the straps don't hang out. Never let your panty lines show.

Knowing how to dress to look slimmer and avoiding making public fashion errors goes a long way in helping build or keep your self-esteem. Look your best, and you'll feel your best.

Even if you're not at your goal weight, there's no reason to hide behind a sweatshirt and baggy pants. Loving your body at any size is what will ultimately make you look great, no matter what you're wearing.

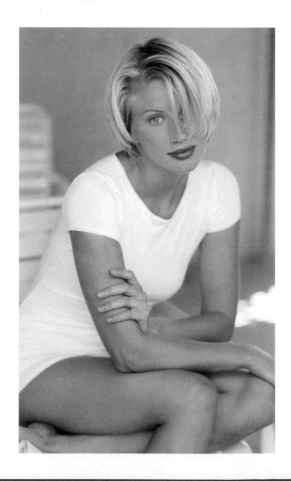

Real People, Real Results.

Challenge:	Start Weight: 224 lbs.
Eliminating unhealthy choices	End Weight: 138 lbs.
	Pounds Lost: 86

Results not typical.

Kristine Got on the Right Track

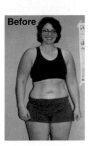
Before

Kristine R. didn't need a calculator to figure out the formula to better health. After linking up with eDiets.com and shedding 86 pounds from her 5-foot, 4-inch frame, she found the answer to success in basic addition and subtraction.

By subtracting poor eating habits and adding a healthy dining regimen, she became a vision of success, shrinking from a snug size 20 to a shape-flattering 10.

The 26-year-old New Yorker had no idea how much fast food and late-night drinking had hurt her health. It wasn't until she saw the number on the scale that she started calculating the repercussions of her lifestyle.

Kristine started by examining her past experiences with dieting. Sure, she lost a few pounds, but she always seemed to gain them right back again. The more she thought about her past trials with weight loss, the more she wanted a different approach.

"I liked that you could just do it from home," Kristine says. "I think it's very hard to go out in public when you weigh a lot.

"The first week or two I didn't lose weight, but then I started losing a little here and a little there, a pound a week, maybe two," she recalls. "After two or three weeks, I started adjusting and getting used to the changes. It was difficult at first, but I knew that if I kept going and doing the right things that the right things would happen.

"Eating wasn't a stigma on my plan. I stopped thinking of food as a regimen and more as an enjoyment, so I just let go a bit and stopped thinking about it all the time. Maintenance is easy. I just eat what's comfortable, listen to myself and know what good choices to make."

She admits that before linking up with eDiets, physical activity had no role in her life. Today, you can catch the new-and-improved Kristine at the gym more days than not.

"I had the strength and the motivation to lose all this weight," she says. "I now feel that I can do just about anything. I am going back to school, and I am much more outgoing."

Six Quotes for
Inspiration

1. "People usually fail when they are on the verge of success. So give as much care to the end as to the beginning."
   – Lao-Tzu

We get all excited and super-committed at the beginning of a new diet. If you just maintain consistency and keep doing what you should, the end will be in sight, and you will realize your dreams and goals! Consistency over time is all you need.

2. "Failure seldom stops you. What stops you is the fear of failure."
   – Jack Lemmon

Fear of failure is the No. 1 reason people don't start a much-needed healthy weight-loss plan!

3. "Victory is won not in miles but in inches. Win a little now, hold your ground, and later, win a little more."
   – Louis L'Amour

This journey is all about inches! Measure your success with each small improvement, each small change and baby step. If you have 50 pounds to lose, each pound lost is a success. Keep an eye on each of your steps and forget about the big picture.

4. "Happiness is when what you think, what you say, and what you do are in harmony."
   – Mahatma Gandhi

Be, do and then you will have! You may pine to be "one of those Whole-Foods-shopping, dog-on-the-beach-walking women." Then get a dog, walk it on the beach, shop at Whole Foods and you will be that woman. You don't suddenly wake up as the ideal you have in mind; you start living the ideal. Quit dreaming; start doing!

5. "The most difficult thing is the decision to act; the rest is merely tenacity."
   – Amelia Earhart

Getting started is the most daunting part of the weight-loss journey. It is easier than you think, so just make the decision and get started!

6. "It takes courage to grow up and turn out to be who you really are."
   – e. e. cummings

Remember that the same person who wants to be like other people they idealize may also be scared to become that person. Don't be afraid – have courage and know that everything is going to work out fine for you as you move down a new and healthful path!

NUTRITION
Tools

The handy nutrition tools in this section will help you make healthy choices whether you're eating at home or on the run.

Nutrition **Facts**

Beverages

Category	Product	Type	Serving Size	Cal	Fat (g)	Carb (g)	Sod (mg)	Prot (g)
Water, Bottled	Perrier		1 cup (8 fl oz)	0	0	0	2.4	0
Coffee	brewed	regular	1 cup (8 fl oz)	0	0	0	2.4	0.2
Juice	orange	canned, unsweetened	1/2 cup	54	0.2	12.3	2.5	0.7
	apple	canned, unsweetened	3/4 cup	87	0.2	21.7	5.6	0.1
	cranberry	100%	1/3 cup	43	0.1	10.3	1.7	0.3
	grapefruit	white, canned, unsweetened	1/2 cup	48	0.1	11.1	1.2	0.6
Milk	milk	1% or low-fat	1 cup (8 fl oz)	102	2.4	12.2	107.4	8.2
		2% or reduced-fat	1 cup (8 fl oz)	121	4.8	11.4	100.0	8.1
		skim	1 cup (8 fl oz)	85	0.4	11.8	126.9	8.3
		whole	1 cup (8 fl oz)	146	7.9	11.0	97.6	7.9
Soft Drinks	cola	caffeinated	1 can (12 fl oz)	160	0	39.8	14.8	0.2
		sugar-free, caffeinated	1 can (12 fl oz)	3	0	0.4	17.8	0.4
		lemon-lime soda	1 can (12 fl oz)	153	0	38.3	40.5	0
		tonic	1 can (12 fl oz)	129	0	32.2	14.6	0
Sport Drinks	energy drink	with caffeine & added vitamins B6 & B12	1 cup (8 fl oz)	112	0	27.0	191.9	1.0
Tea	instant	unsweeted with lemon	1 cup (8 fl oz)	4	0	1.0	14.3	0
		caffeinated, sugar & lemon	1 cup (8 fl oz)	90	0.1	22.1	7.8	0.1
Alcoholic Beverages	beer	regular	1 can (12 fl oz)	139	0	10.8	14.2	1.1
		light	1 can (12 fl oz)	103	0	5.2	14.2	1.0
	wine	red	1 fl oz	21	0	0.5	1.5	0.1
		white	1 fl oz	20	0	0.2	1.5	0
	martini		1 fl oz	30	0	0.6	0.8	0

Bread & Baked Goods

Category	Product	Type	Serving Size	Cal	Fat (g)	Carb (g)	Sod (mg)	Prot (g)
Specialty Breads	bagel	egg	1 bagel (4" dia)	287	2.2	55.7	530.3	11.1
		cinnamon-raisin	1 bagel (4" dia)	245	1.5	49.1	286.6	8.7
	croissant	cheese	1 medium	235	11.9	26.8	316.3	5.2
	pita	white	1 small (4" dia)	77	0.3	15.6	150.1	2.5
Breads	breadstick	plain	1 stick	41	1.0	6.8	65.7	1.2
	garlic bread		1 piece	186	9.6	20.8	200.0	4.2
	wheat bread	whole	1 slice	69	1.2	12.9	147.6	2.7
		bran	1 slice	93	1.2	17.2	175.0	3.2
Crackers	cheese cracker	regular	1/2 cup	155	7.8	18.0	308.5	3.1
	Wasa bread		1 piece	31	0.1	7.0	22.4	0.7
	Ritz cracker		5 crackers	79	3.7	10.3	124.2	1.2
	Snackwell cracker	pepper	1 cracker	4	0.1	0.7	7.3	0.1
Pancakes & Waffles	pancake	frozen	1 pancake	81	1.2	15.4	256.6	2.2
	waffle	frozen, plain	1 waffle	160	5.0	29.0	390.0	5.0
Rolls	English muffin		1 muffin	155	1.9	31.1	135.9	7.8
	hamburger or hot dog bun	plain	1 bun	118	1.9	21.3	206.0	4.1
Tortillas & Tacos	taco shell		1 shell	62	3.0	8.3	48.8	1.0
	tortilla	corn	1 medium	53	0.6	11.2	38.6	1.4
		flour	1 tortilla	104	2.3	17.8	153.0	2.8
Quick Bread	banana bread	homemade with margarine	1 slice	198	6.3	32.8	181.2	2.6
	pizza dough		1 oz	75	1.0	13.4	189.0	2.5
	cornbread	prepared from mix	1 piece	187	6.0	28.9	466.8	4.3

Breakfast Cereals

Category	Product	Type	Serving Size	Cal	Fat (g)	Carb (g)	Sod (mg)	Prot (g)
Cold	All-Bran		1 cup	156	2.0	44.4	154.8	7.5
	Cheerios		1 cup	81	1.8	22.2	273.0	3.3
	Corn Flakes		1 cup	106	0.2	24.1	203.0	2.0
	Muesli	dried fruit and nuts	1 cup	335	4.2	66.1	196.4	8.2
	Special K		1 cup	120	0.5	22.0	223.5	7.0
Hot	oatmeal	instant	1 packet	103	1.7	17.9	80.1	4.3
	Cream of Wheat	instant with salt, prepared with water	1/2 cup	75	0.3	15.8	182.0	2.2
		regular with salt, cooked with water	1/2 cup	63	0.2	13.5	168.2	1.8
	Roman Meal	plain with salt, cooked with water	1/2 cup	83	0.5	16.5	98.8	3.3

Nutrition Bars & Products

Category	Product	Type	Serving Size	Cal	Fat (g)	Carb (g)	Sod (mg)	Prot (g)
	AdvantEdge	carb-control	1 bar	200	7.0	21.0	125.0	24.0
		carb-control crisp	1 bar	230	7.0	27.0	350.0	20.0
		chewy	1 bar	210	5.0	27.0	160.0	15.0
		crispy	1 bar	210	5.0	27.0	160.0	15.0
		Morning Energy	1 bar	170	6.0	22.0	100.0	11.0
		SoNutty	1 bar	210	8.0	18.0	120.0	15.0
	Atkins	Advantage	1 bar	230	11.0	11.0	100.0	19.0
		Advantage granola	1 bar	200	9.0	17.0	150.0	17.0
		Endulge candy, chocolate-covered	1 bar	180	12.0	20.0	70.0	4.0
		Endulge candy, chocolate-peanut or chocolate-almond	1 bar	220	10.0	24.0	200.0	9.0
		Endulge candy, chocolate-raspberry	1 bar	150	12.0	16.0	5.0	1.0
		Morning Start breakfast	1 bar	170	9.0	13.0	70.0	11.0
		Morning Start fruit & grain cereal	1 bar	100	2.0	20.0	74.9	5.0
	Choice_DM	Berry Almond Crispy	1 bar	50	1.0	10.0	25.0	2.0
		Chocolate Peanut Butter Crispy	1 bar	60	2.0	10.0	35.0	1.0
		Fudge Brownie Nutrition	1 bar	140	4.5	19.0	80.0	6.0
		Lemon-Lime Fiber-Bust	1 bar	45	1.0	12.0	0	1.0
		Peanutty Chocolate Nutrition Bar	1 bar	140	4.5	19.0	80.0	6.0
		Tropical Fruit Fiber-Bust	1 bar	45	1.0	11.0	0	1.0
	Power Bars	Performance	1 bar	230	2.0	45.0	100.0	9.0
		Pria	1 bar	110	3.0	16.0	80.0	5.0
		Pria Carb Select	1 bar	130	6.0	16.0	140.0	8.0
	Slim-Fast	Chewy Granola	1 bar	220	5.0	35.0	250.0	8.0
		Low-Carb Diet Meal	1 bar	200	8.0	17.0	240.0	16.0
		Low-Carb Diet Snack	1 bar	120	3.0	18.0	80.0	6.0
		Layered Meal	1 bar	220	5.0	34.0	160.0	8.0
		Meal On-The-Go	1 bar	220	5.0	35.0	140.0	8.0
		Snack	1 bar	120	4.0	21.0	75.0	1.0
		Low-Carb Diet Breakfast	1 bar	180	5.0	18.0	279.7	14.0
		Optima Breakfast	1 bar	180	6.0	22.0	200.0	10.0
		Optima Chewy Granola Meal	1 bar	220	5.0	34.0	300.0	8.0
		Optima Cookies Snack	1 bar	120	3.5	19.0	110.0	2.0
		Optima Meal	1 bar	220	5.0	35.0	160.0	8.0

Nutrition Bars & Products

Category	Product	Type	Serving Size	Cal	Fat (g)	Carb (g)	Sod (mg)	Prot (g)
	Slim-Fast	Optima Muffin	1 bar	140	5.0	22.0	170.0	1.0
		Optima Snack	1 bar	120	4.0	20.0	70.0	2.0
	Body for Life	assorted flavors	1 bar	200	7.0	21.0	250.0	15.0
	Clif Bars	Apricot	1 bar	230	3.0	46.0	90.0	10.0
		Black Cherry	1 bar	230	5.0	44.0	110.0	10.0
		Carrot Cake	1 bar	240	4.0	46.0	150.0	10.0
		Chocolate Almond Fudge	1 bar	250	5.0	44.0	140.0	10.0
		Chocolate Brownie	1 bar	240	4.5	45.0	150.0	10.0
		Chocolate Chip	1 bar	250	5.0	45.0	150.0	10.0
		Chocolate Chip Peanut Crunch	1 bar	250	6.0	43.0	210.0	11.0
		Cookies 'N Cream	1 bar	240	4.0	47.0	180.0	10.0
		Cool Mint Chocolate	1 bar	250	5.0	43.0	140.0	10.0
		Cranberry Apple	1 bar	230	2.5	45.0	100.0	10.0
		Crunchy Peanut Butter	1 bar	250	6.0	40.0	250.0	12.0
		Lemon Poppyseed	1 bar	230	3.5	46.0	110.0	10.0
		Oatmeal Raisin Walnut	1 bar	245	5.0	43.0	125.0	10.0
		Peanut Toffee Buzz	1 bar	250	6.0	42.0	200.0	11.0
	Kashi GOLEAN Crunchy!	Chocolate Caramel Karma	1 bar	140	3.0	26.0	180.0	8.0
		Chocolate Peanut Bliss	1 bar	170	4.0	30.0	220.0	9.0
		Sublime Lemon-Lime	1 bar	160	3.0	32.0	150.0	9.0
	Kashi GOLEAN Original	Chocolate Almond Toffee	1 bar	290	6.0	45.0	250.0	13.0
		Cookies 'N' Cream	1 bar	290	6.0	50.0	200.0	13.0
		Frosted Spice Cake	1 bar	290	5.0	49.0	200.0	13.0
		Honey Vanilla Yogurt	1 bar	290	5.0	49.0	160.0	13.0
		Malted Chocolate Crisp	1 bar	290	6.0	49.0	200.0	13.0
		Mocha Java	1 bar	290	6.0	50.0	190.0	13.0
		Oatmeal Raisin Cookies	1 bar	280	5.0	49.0	140.0	13.0
		Peanut Butter & Chocolate	1 bar	290	6.0	48.0	280.0	13.0
		Strawberries 'N' Cream	1 bar	290	5.0	50.0	200.0	13.0
	Luna	Caramel Apple	1 bar	170	2.0	29.0	160.0	10.0
		Cherry-Covered Chocolate	1 bar	180	4.0	28.0	140.0	10.0
		Chocolate Peppermint	1 bar	180	4.0	29.0	130.0	10.0
		Dulce de Leche	1 bar	180	2.5	29.0	160.0	10.0
		Key Lime Pie	1 bar	180	4.0	29.0	80.0	10.0
		Lemonzest	1 bar	180	4.0	26.0	50.0	10.0
		Nutz Over Chocolate	1 bar	180	4.5	24.0	100.0	10.0
		Orange Bliss	1 bar	180	4.0	29.0	100.0	10.0
		Peanut Butter 'N' Jelly	1 bar	170	2.5	28.0	190.0	10.0
		S'Mores	1 bar	180	4.5	26.0	125.0	10.0
		Sesame Raisin Crunch	1 bar	170	3.0	26.0	125.0	10.0
		Sweet Dreams	1 bar	180	4.0	27.0	160.0	10.0
		Toasted Nuts 'N' Cranberry	1 bar	170	3.0	26.0	130.0	10.0
		Tropical Crisp	1 bar	180	4.5	24.0	135.0	10.0

Convenience Foods

Category	Product	Type	Serving Size	Cal	Fat (g)	Carb (g)	Sod (mg)	Prot (g)
Frozen Foods	Budget Gourmet	Italian sausage lasagna	1 package	457	23.8	39.9	902.9	20.6
	Gorton's frozen fish	grilled salmon fillet	1 fillet	100	3.0	0	380.0	17.0
	Healthy Choice	beef pot roast	1 package	320	9.0	39.0	550.0	19.0
	Lean Cuisine	roasted turkey & vegetables	1 package	150	5.0	12.0	650.0	15.0

Convenience Foods

Category	Product	Type	Serving Size	Cal	Fat (g)	Carb (g)	Sod (mg)	Prot (g)
Packaged Foods	Hamburger Helper	cheeseburger macaroni, dry mix	1 serving	178	4.7	28.9	913.5	5.0
	instant potatoes	flakes	1/2 cup	25	0	5.5	6.0	0.5
	Kraft Mac & Cheese	NLEA serving	1 cup prep.	259	2.6	47.5	561.4	11.3
Frozen Pizza	pepperoni		1 serving	400	21.1	36.2	878.9	16.2
	Celeste	sausage, peppers & mushrooms	1 serving	386	20.7	33.2	764.9	16.7

Fast Foods

Category	Product	Type	Serving Size	Cal	Fat (g)	Carb (g)	Sod (mg)	Prot (g)
McDonald's	Big Mac		each	600	33.0	50.0	1010.0	25.0
	Quarter Pounder	with cheese	each	540	29.0	39.0	1150.0	29.0
	French Fries	medium	each	350	16.0	47.0	220.0	4.0
	McChicken		each	420	22.0	41.0	760.0	15.0
	Bacon Ranch Salad	with grilled chicken	each	240	9.0	11.0	940.0	31.0
Burger King	Whopper		each	700	42.0	52.0	1020.0	31.0
	French Fries	medium	each	360	18.0	46.0	640.0	4.0
	Chicken Tenders		1 tender	42	2.4	2.6	0	2.8
	Caesar Salad	fire-grilled chicken	each	190	7.0	9.0	900.0	25.0
Wendy's	Classic Single		each	410	19.0	37.0	0	25.0
	Big Bacon Classic		each	580	29.0	45.0	0	33.0
	French Fries	medium	each	390	17.0	56.0	340.0	4.0
	Mandarin Chicken Salad	no almonds or rice noodes	each	170	3.0	17.0	740.0	22.0
	Frosty	small	12 oz.	330	8.0	56.0	150.0	8.0
Starbucks	coffee Frappuccino	blended coffee	grande	260	3.5	52.0	250.0	5.0
	blueberry muffin		1 muffin	380	19.0	49.0	380.0	5.0
Subway	tuna wrap	with cheese	each	440	32.0	16.0	1310.0	27.0
	roasted chicken breast salad		each	125	3.0	8.0	615.0	16.0
	cold cut combo	6-inch	each	410	17.0	46.0	0	23.0
	turkey breast, ham & bacon	6-inch	each	380	12.0	47.0	0	25.0
Taco Bell	taco	beef, soft	each	210	10.0	21.0	0	10.0
	quesadilla	cheese	each	490	28.0	39.0	0	19.0
	burrito	supreme, beef	each	440	18.0	51.0	1330.0	18.0
	bowl	Zesty chicken	each	550	17.0	62.0	0	21.0

Salad Dressings & Oils

Category	Product	Type	Serving Size	Cal	Fat (g)	Carb (g)	Sod (mg)	Prot (g)
Oil	corn		1 tsp	41	4.5	0	0	0
	olive		1 tsp	40	4.5	0	0.1	0
Butter	salted		1 tsp	35	3.8	0	27.2	0
Margarine	low or nonfat		1 tsp	2	0	0	29.6	0
Mayonnaise	regular		1 tsp	100	11.0	0	75.0	0
Salad Dressings	Caesar		1 tsp	54	5.4	0.5	142.1	0.5
	Italian		1 tsp	44	4.2	1.5	243.1	0.1
	oil & vinegar	homemade	1 tsp	74	8.0	0.4	0.2	0
	coleslaw dressing		1 tsp	64	5.3	3.8	113.6	0.1

Fish

Category	Product	Type	Serving Size	Cal	Fat (g)	Carb (g)	Sod (mg)	Prot (g)
Canned	salmon	regular	1 oz	40	1.6	0	138.1	6.1
	shrimp		1 oz	34	0.6	0.3	47.9	6.5
	tuna	white, in water	1 oz	36	0.8	0	106.9	6.7
Sushi	small roll	avocado	each	18	0.4	3.2	11.0	0.3
		cucumber	each	14	0	3.1	10.8	0.3
Finfish	cod		1 oz	23	0.2	0	15.3	5.0
	grouper	baked or broiled	1 oz	31	0.4	0	15.0	7.0
	whitefish	smoked	1 oz, boneless	29	0.3	0	288.9	6.6
Other Fish	surimi	imitation crab or loster	1 oz	27	0.3	1.9	40.5	4.3
	bluefish		1 oz	35	1.2	0	17.0	5.7

Fruit & Juices

Category	Product	Type	Serving Size	Cal	Fat (g)	Carb (g)	Sod (mg)	Prot (g)
Fruits	apple	medium	2-3/4" dia	72	0.2	19.1	1.4	0.4
	banana	raw	1 small (4oz)	101	0.4	25.9	1.1	1.2
	mango	fresh	1/2 cup	54	0.2	14.0	1.7	0.4
	nectarine		1 small (2-1/2" dia)	67	0.4	14.3	0	1.4
	orange	all varieties	1 small (2-3/8" dia)	45	0.1	11.3	0	0.9
Citrus Juices	grapefruit	pink, fresh	1/2 cup	49	0.1	11.4	1.2	0.6
		white, canned, unsweeted	1/2 cup	48	0.1	11.1	1.2	0.6
	orange	canned, unsweeted	1/2 cup	54	0.2	12.3	2.5	0.7
	pineapple	canned, unsweeted	1/2 cup	70	0.1	17.2	1.3	0.4

Meats

Category	Product	Type	Serving Size	Cal	Fat (g)	Carb (g)	Sod (mg)	Prot (g)
Beef	corned beef	with potato, canned	1/2 cup	212	13.2	12.0	548.3	11.31
	steak	chuck - broiled, extra lean	1 oz	43	1.6	0	20.1	7.3
	ground beef	regular, broiled	1 oz	77	5.3	0	22.1	7.2
	ribs	roasted beef	1 oz	114	9.8	0	17.9	6.3
Pork	bacon	baked	1 slice cooked	44	3.5	0.1	177.6	2.9
	pork chops	pan-fried, bone-in	1 oz	73	4.8	0	14.2	7.5
	breakfast strips	cooked	1 slice cooked	51	4.1	0.1	237.2	3.3
	ham	boneless, roasted, regular smoked or cured,	1 oz	49	2.6	0	425.3	6.4
		lean, cooked	1 oz	39	1.6	0.4	274.7	5.9
Veal	ground	broiled	1 oz	47	2.1	0	23.5	6.9
	loin chop	roasted	1 oz	60	3.5	0	26.4	7.0
Lamb	chop	lean	1 oz	41	1.7	0	19.3	5.9
	hocks	braised	1 oz	67	3.8	0	20.4	8.0

Pasta & Grains

Category	Product	Type	Serving Size	Cal	Fat (g)	Carb (g)	Sod (mg)	Prot (g)
Pasta	macaroni	cooked	1/3 cup	65	0.3	13.3	0.5	2.2
	spaghetti	cooked with salt	1/3 cup	65	0.3	13.2	46.6	2.2
	ravioli	light, refrigerated	1/3 cup	94	2.4	13.4	133.1	5.0
	noodles	Japanese somen, cooked	1/3 cup	75	0.1	16.1	94.3	2.3

Rice & Cooked Grains

Category	Product	Type	Serving Size	Cal	Fat (g)	Carb (g)	Sod (mg)	Prot (g)
	white rice	instant, long grain, cooked	1/3 cup	52	0.1	11.7	1.7	1.1
	brown rice	long grain, cooked	1/3 cup	72	0.6	14.9	3.3	1.7
	couscous	cooked	1/3 cup	57	0.1	12.1	2.6	2.0

Poultry

Category	Product	Type	Serving Size	Cal	Fat (g)	Carb (g)	Sod (mg)	Prot (g)
Chicken	capon	roasted, with skin	1 oz	63	3.3	0	13.9	8.2
	wings	meat and skin, stewed	1 oz	69	4.8	0	19.0	6.5
	canned		1 oz	30	0.5	0.5	114.4	5.5
Duck	roasted	no skin	1 oz	55	3.2	0	18.4	6.7
Turkey	patty	breaded, battered, fried	1 oz	264	16.9	14.8	752.0	13.2
	smoked	with skin	1 oz	46	1.4	0	282.4	8.3
	ground	cooked	1 oz	67	3.7	0	30.3	7.8

Lunch & Deli Meats

Category	Product	Type	Serving Size	Cal	Fat (g)	Carb (g)	Sod (mg)	Prot (g)
Chicken Breast	cooked and sliced	low-sodium	1 oz	26	0	2.0	244.9	5.1
Turkey	white rotisserie	deli-cut	1 oz	32	0.9	2.2	340.2	3.8
	turkey breast	regular	1 slice	28	0.5	1.2	284.2	4.8
	turkey roll	light and dark meat	1 slice	41	2.0	0.6	166.1	5.1
	turkey ham	prepackaged or deli-cut, extra lean	1 oz	34	1.1	0.4	294.3	5.6

Soups

Category	Product	Type	Serving Size	Cal	Fat (g)	Carb (g)	Sod (mg)	Prot (g)
	bean	black bean	1 cup (8 fl oz)	54	0.5	10.7	282.2	2.9
	cream of mushroom	ready-to-serve	1 can (10.75 oz)	329	21.9	26.9	118.6	5.9
	chicken broth	canned	1 cup (8 fl oz)	35	1.4	0.9	763.2	4.8
	chicken noodle		1 cup (8 fl oz)	120	2.0	19.0	480.0	8.0
	gazpacho	ready-to-serve	1 cup (8 fl oz)	48	0.2	4.4	739.3	7.1
	onion	mix	1 Tbsp	20	0	5.0	530.0	0
	tomato	prepared with water	1 cup (8 fl oz)	92	1.9	16.6	695.4	2.0
	vegetable	broth	1 cup (8 fl oz)	30	0.5	5.0	460.0	1.0

Snacks

Category	Product	Type	Serving Size	Cal	Fat (g)	Carb (g)	Sod (mg)	Prot (g)
Breakfast & Snack Bars	Nutri-Grain cereal bars	mixed berry	1 bar	139	2.8	26.9	109.9	1.6
		fruit-flavored	1 bar	139	2.8	27.0	109.9	1.6
	crisped rice bar	chocolate chip	1 bar	121	3.8	20.4	77.8	1.4
	Special K	blueberry	each	90	1.5	18.0	85.0	2.0
		cranberry apple	each	90	2.0	17.0	90.0	2.0

Snacks

Category	Product	Type	Serving Size	Cal	Fat (g)	Carb (g)	Sod (mg)	Prot (g)
Chips & Salty Snacks	beef sticks	smoked	1 oz	157	14.1	1.5	419.6	6.1
	popcorn	microwave, low fat and sodium	1 cup	25	0.6	4.3	28.4	0.7
		caramel-coated	1 oz	127	3.6	22.4	58.4	1.1
	potato chips	plain, salted	1 oz	156	9.8	15.0	168.4	2.0
		sour cream & onion	1 oz	154	9.6	14.6	177.2	2.3
	tortilla chips	regular, unsalted	1 oz	67	3.4	8.2	31.5	1.0
Salsa	tomatoes		1/2 cup	42	0.3	8.1	562.0	1.6

Sweets & Treats

Category	Product	Type	Serving Size	Cal	Fat (g)	Carb (g)	Sod (mg)	Prot (g)
	brownies	homemade	2" square	117	7	12	82.3	1.5
		Little Debbie, ready-to-eat	1 package (twin)	257	9.9	39.0	190.3	2.9
	cookies	chocolate chip, ready-to-eat	1 medium, 2.5"	49	2.3	6.7	31.5	0.5
	ice cream	chocolate, regular	1 cup	150	7.3	18.6	50.2	2.5
		strawberry	1 cup	131	5.5	18.2	39.6	2.1
		vanilla, regular	1/3 cup	299	15.8	34.0	115.2	5.0
	pudding	rice, made with 2% milk	1/2 cup	126	1.9	23.5	123.7	3.7
	chewing gum	regular	1 stick	8	0	2.0	0	0
	candy	M&M's, Mars, Snickers	1 bar (2 oz)	279	14.0	33.7	151.6	4.6

Vegetables

Category	Product	Type	Serving Size	Cal	Fat (g)	Carb (g)	Sod (mg)	Prot (g)
Potatoes	boiled	no skin	1/2 cup	68	0.1	15.6	3.9	1.3
	french fries	frozen, with salt	10 pieces	92	3.4	14.0	119.7	1.4
	mashed	instant, with whole milk and margarine	1/2 cup	124	5.9	15.8	348.6	2.0
Vegetables	green beans	frozen	1 cup	25	0	5.0	95.0	1.0
	carrots	boiled, with salt	1/2 cup	29	0.1	6.4	235.6	0.6
	peas	canned	1/2 cup	60	0.3	10.7	214.2	3.8
Tomatoes	raw	medium	1 cup	25	0.4	5.6	10.8	1.0
	sauce	regular	1/2 cup	39	0.3	9.0	641.9	1.6
Prepared Vegetables	coleslaw	homemade	1/2 cup	47	1.6	7.4	13.8	0.8
	potato salad	homemade	1/2 cup	162	10.3	14.0	661.3	3.4
	onion rings	breaded	1/2 cup	99	6.4	9.2	90.0	1.3
	spinach souffle	homemade	1 cup	221	18.4	2.8	763.0	11.0
Vegetables, Cooked	broccoli	boiled, with salt	1/2 cup	28	0.3	3.9	204.4	2.3
	green pepper	sweet, sauteed	1/2 cup	94	8.8	3.1	12.7	0.6
	squash	summer, all varieties, boiled, with salt	1 cup	56	0.4	10.6	464.6	2.5
Vegetables, Raw	avocado	all varieties	2 Tbsp	48	4.6	2.2	3.0	0.6
	asparagus		1/2 cup	17	0.1	2.6	1.3	1.5
	onion	sweet	1 cup	55	0.1	12.1	12.8	1.3
	garlic		1 tsp	4	0	0.9	0.5	0.2

Source: eDiets.com® Nutrition Tracker™ - Use Nutrition Tracker free at www.eDiets.com.

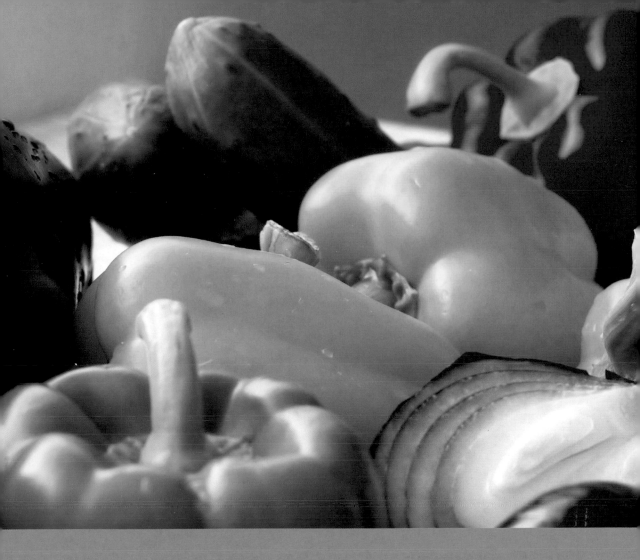

Substitution **Guide**

This guide shows you how to exchange one food for another. All foods within the same category are interchangeable. Just follow the serving sizes.

▷ Breads:

- 1 slice regular bread
- 2 slices 40-calorie diet bread
- 1/2 small bagel (3 oz. bagel)
- 1/2 English muffin
- 1/2 hamburger or hot dog bun
- 1/2 pita bread (6-inch)
- 2 Wasa Light Bread
- 4 Melba Toast
- 6 saltine crackers
- 2 rice cakes (4-inch, 35 calories each)
- 1 tortilla (corn or flour, 6 to 8-inch)
- 2 low-fat pancakes (4-inch)
- 1 low-fat waffle (4-inch)
- 1 slice low-fat French toast
- 1 board of matzo (1 oz.)

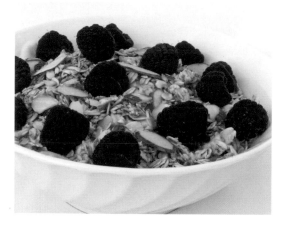

▷ Cereals, Grains & Pasta

- 3/4 cup flaked or Chex-type cereal
- 1 1/2 cup puffed cereal (wheat or rice)
- 1/2 cup cooked hot cereal
- 1/3 cup nugget-type cereal (Grape-Nuts)
- 1/4 cup low-fat granola
- 1/2 cup cooked kasha, millet, grits, barley, or couscous
- 1/2 cup pasta, cooked
- 1/3 cup white or brown rice, cooked
- 1 oz. Wheat Germ (4 Tbsp.)

▷ Starchy Vegetables

- 1 small or 1/2 medium potato
- 1 small or 1/2 medium sweet potato
- 1/2 cup mashed potatoes
- 1 cup winter squash (butternut or acorn)
- 1/2 cup cooked plantain or cassava
- 1/2 cup cooked corn
- 1 small piece corn on the cob
- 2/3 cup lima beans, cooked
- 1/3 cup baked beans
- 1/2 cup dried beans and peas, cooked
- 1/2 cup lentils, split peas, or black-eyed peas, cooked
- 1/2 cup soybeans, cooked
- 1/2 cup green peas

▷ Meat & Meat Substitutes

- 1 oz. lean meat, veal or pork
- 1 oz. skinless poultry
- 1 oz. game meat
- 1 oz. fish
- 1 oz. shellfish
- 1 oz. water-packed tuna, salmon or sardines
- 1 oz. low-fat sausage or turkey sausage
- 1 whole egg
- 2 egg whites
- 1/4 cup egg replacement
- 1/4 cup nonfat or low-fat cottage cheese
- 1/3 cup nonfat or low-fat ricotta cheese
- 1 oz. low-fat or nonfat cheese
- 2 Tbsp. grated Parmesan cheese
- 1 slice luncheon meat
- 1 oz. tofu or 2 oz. low-fat tofu
- 1 oz. tempeh (soybean cake)
- 1 vegetarian burger = 2 oz. lean meat

▷ Milk & Milk Substitutes

- 1 cup low-fat (1%) or nonfat (skim) milk
- 1 cup low-fat or nonfat buttermilk
- 1/2 cup evaporated nonfat milk
- 1/3 cup dry nonfat milk

- 1 cup low-fat or nonfat soy yogurt
- 1 cup pudding made with nonfat milk
- 1 cup low-fat or nonfat yogurt
- 1 cup low-fat or nonfat soy milk
- 1 cup low-fat or nonfat rice milk
- 1 cup low-fat or nonfat Lactaid milk
- 1 cup low-fat or nonfat almond milk
- 1 cup low-fat or nonfat oat milk

▷ Fruit

- 1 small apple, orange, peach or pear
- 1 cup cubed melon
- 1 cup berries
- 1/2 medium banana
- 17 small grapes
- 12 sweet fresh cherries
- 1/2 large grapefruit
- 4 oz. fruit juice
- 1/2 cup canned fruit in juice or water
- 1 kiwi fruit
- 2 Tbsp. raisins
- 4 dried prunes
- 5 dried apple rings
- 4 apricot halves

▷ Salads & Vegetables

1 cup raw or 1/2 cup cooked:
- artichokes, asparagus
- beans (green, snap), beets, broccoli, Brussels sprouts
- cabbage, carrots, cauliflower, celery, collards, cucumber, chives
- dandelion greens
- eggplant, endive, escarole
- fennel
- garlic
- horseradish
- jicama
- kale, kohlrabi
- leeks, lettuce
- mushrooms, mustard greens

- okra, onions
- peppers, parsley, pea pods
- radishes
- seaweed, snow peas, spinach, summer squash, sorrel, shallot, sprouts
- tomatoes
- watercress, water chestnuts
- zucchini

▷ Fats

- 1 tsp. butter
- 1 tsp. oil
- 1 tsp. margarine or mayonnaise
- 1 Tbsp. light butter or mayonnaise
- 1 tsp. salad dressing
- 1 Tbsp. light dressing
- 2 tsp. peanut butter
- 1 Tbsp. cream cheese
- 2 Tbsp. reduced-fat cream cheese
- 3 Tbsp. nonfat cream cheese
- 1 Tbsp. sour cream
- 3 Tbsp. low-fat sour cream
- 8 olives
- 1 oz. avocado
- 6 almonds or cashews
- 10 peanuts
- 4 pecan halves
- 1 Tbsp. sesame seeds
- 1 Tbsp. sunflower seeds

▷ Free Foods

- low-sodium bouillon or broth
- sugar-free drinks, club soda or seltzer
- herbal or decaffeinated tea or coffee
- sugar-free gelatin (3 servings daily)
- sugar-free chewing gum (5 sticks daily)
- nonfat sugar-free whipped topping (2 Tbsp.)
- vinegar, lemon and lime juice
- ketchup, horseradish, mustard, dill pickles
- raw salad (unlimited)
- non-stick cooking spray

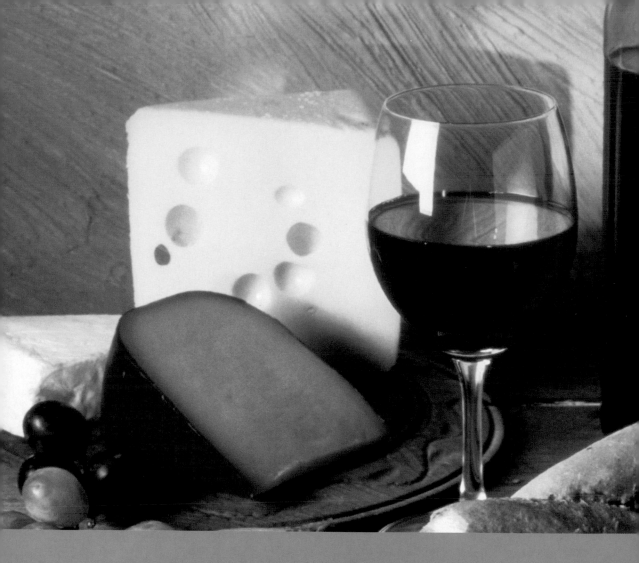

Dining Out **Guide**

Dining out doesn't have to wreck your diet.
Use these guidelines to help you make healthy
choices wherever you may be.

▷ Bagels:

- Choose plain, whole-wheat, sesame or pumpernickel.
- Use reduced-fat cream cheese or jam.
- "Scoop out" your bagel.

▷ Barbeque:

- Order barbeque sauce on the side.
- Pass on the ribs.
- Order chicken breast, fish or pork tenderloin.

▷ Beverages:

- Skip the soda, sweet tea, fruit drinks and sports drinks.
- Choose sparkling water or diet soda.
- Enjoy tea, coffee or a latte with low-fat or fat-free milk.
- Choose fat-free, low-fat or reduced-fat milk.

▷ Breakfast:

- A buttermilk pancake is better than a waffle. Choose light or sugar-free syrup.
- Order hot cereal with fat-free milk.
- Choose Canadian bacon instead of sausage, bacon or ham.
- Make French toast with egg whites. Spray skillet with cooking spray.
- Hold the butter!

▷ Buffet:

- Skip the high-fat salad dressings, croutons, olives and sunflower seeds.
- Pass on egg, chicken and tuna salads made with full-fat mayonnaise.
- Fill up on salads and fresh veggies.
- Skip the dips and spreads.
- Baked ham, turkey, chicken, fish and shrimp are good choices.

▷ Chicken:

- Roasted or rotisserie is best. Remove skin.
- Skip the mayo on a chicken sandwich.
- Choose baked, boiled or grilled, not fried.
- White meat is healthier than dark meat.

▷ Chinese:

- Avoid dishes named "crispy," "sweet and sour" and "bird's nest."
- Skip the egg rolls, spare ribs, chow mien and chop suey.
- Start your meal with hot and sour, wonton or egg drop soup.
- Choose white rice instead of fried rice.
- Dim sum is a good choice, but order it steamed.
- Choose fresh fruit or a fortune cookie for dessert.
- Order stir-fry items "light on the oil" or ask the chef to stir-fry your meal in broth.

▷ Deli:

- Choose turkey, chicken, roast beef or ham over corned beef and pastrami.
- Ketchup and mustard are fine, but skip the mayo unless it's low-fat.
- Add lettuce and tomato to sandwiches for more fiber.
- Pickles are low in calories, but high in sodium.
- Pass on the hot dogs. They are high in fat, sodium and nitrates.
- Share your sandwich, or save half for tomorrow.
- Skip the side salads made with full-fat mayonnaise.
- Vegetable or bean soups are good choices
- Choose whole grain breads.
- Scoop our your sub roll or bun to save calories.

▷ Fast Food:

- Choose a side salad with low-fat dressing instead of fries.
- Never super-size!
- On a burger, hold the cheese, bacon and special sauce.
- McDonald's fruit and yogurt parfait is a low-calorie, low-fat option.
- Wendy's Garden Sensation Salads aren't so sensational for your diet.
- Order chicken sandwiches grilled and skip the mayo.
- Order your subs with no mayo or oil. Scoop out your sub roll.
- At Arby's, order Roast Chicken Deluxe or Roast Turkey Deluxe without the mayo.

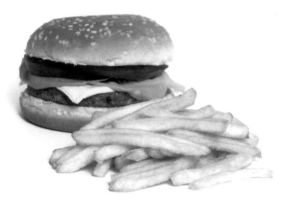

- Fried fish is worse than a hamburger.
- Subway has seven sandwiches with less than 300 calories and six grams of fat.
- Wendy's baked potatoes are good, but skip the sour cream, cheese, bacon and butter.
- Skip high-fat pizza toppings like sausage and pepperoni, and pile on the veggies!
- At Taco Bell, choose a soft taco or a light chicken burrito.

▷ French:

- Skip the escargot and pâté.
- Start with consommé, bouillabaisse or a small salad.
- Foie Gras is not diet-friendly.
- Avoid butter and heavy sauces, like Bearnaise sauce.
- Coquilles Saint-Jacques is a healthy choice.
- Avoid lamb and duck.

▷ Greek:

- Souvlaki, kebabs and skewered meats with vegetables are good choices.
- Order Greek salad without feta cheese and olives.
- Gyros can have more than 700 calories and 40 grams of fat!
- Spanokopita is high in fat.
- Tabouli is a light, healthy option.

▷ Ice Cream:

- Order a small low-fat ice cream or soft-serve low-fat frozen yogurt.
- Order smoothies made with fat-free milk or low-fat frozen yogurt.
- Sorbet is low-calorie and fat-free.
- Skip the toppings!

▷ Indian:

- Tandoori is a safe bet.
- Mango Lassi is not a low-calorie option.
- Mulligatawny is high in saturated fat.
- Order dishes without "ghee."
- Pullao is a low-fat side dish.
- Samosas and Raita are not diet-friendly.

▷ Italian:

- Start your meal with salad. Choose a low-fat dressing, or dress your salad with olive oil and vinegar.
- Select chicken and fish entrees that are grilled, broiled or poached in wine.

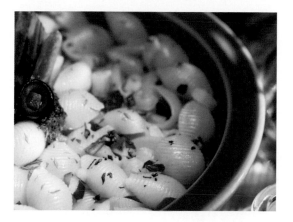

- Avoid lasagna and cheese-filled noodles.
- Order pasta in an appetizer-size portion.
- Avoid cream and butter sauces.
- Choose marinara or pomodoro sauce.
- Avoid dishes with the words "Alfredo," "Bolognese," "Carbonara" and "Parmesan" in their names.
- Watch your portion sizes.
- For dessert, choose espresso, fresh fruit or sorbet.

▷ Japanese:

- Avoid tempura-style dishes and deep-fried dumplings.
- Ebi-su, Miso soup, Edamame, Ohitashi seaweed salad, Oshinko, Shumai, Yakitori, Yaki-udon and Yutofu are healthy choices.
- Maguro, Tako, Saba, Ika, Ebi and Sake Sashimi are good choices.
- Avoid sushi drizzled with eel sauce.
- Choose California rolls or Maki rolls.
- Choose an entrée with steamed vegetables and rice, like Shabu-shabu.
- Yosenabe, Yakitori, Yakimono and Teriyaki chicken are good choices.
- Green tea is rich in cancer-protecting antioxidants.

▷ Mexican:

- Low-fat salsa, gazpacho, beans and corn tortillas are good choices.
- Salsa is fine, but the fried chips are high in fat and calories.
- Pass on sour cream and shredded cheese and limit guacamole.
- Avoid hard taco shells, nachos, quesadillas and refried beans.
- Arroz con pollo, camarones, fajitas and mole de pollo are good choices.

▷ Salad:

- Avoid croutons and bacon bits, marinated veggies and regular salad dressings.
- A Caesar salad is filled with fat.

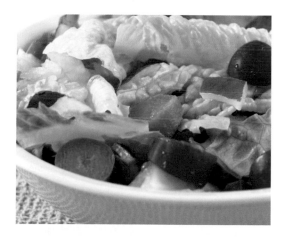

▷ Seafood:

- Order fish, shrimp and shellfish broiled, baked or grilled, not fried.
- Avoid butter and cream sauces.

▷ Side Dishes:

- Avoid fried side dishes.
- Order a plain baked potato.
- Skip high-fat sides like potato salad and coleslaw.
- Skip high-calorie biscuits and baked beans.
- Order corn on the cob or vegetables without butter.

▷ Sporting Events & Outings:

- A small hot dog has 250 calories. Stop at one and skip the fries.
- One serving of nachos has 700 calories.
- Soft pretzels have 200 calories.
- The smallest concession-stand soda has 250 calories. Drink water instead.

▷ Steak House:

- Avoid "stuffed," fried and sauteed dishes.
- Portions are huge. Share with a friend.
- Order the smallest, leanest cut of steak (loin or round).

▷ Subs & Sandwiches:

- Pile on the lettuce, tomato, onions and veggies, but hold the mayo.
- Choose pita or whole-grain breads, or scoop out your sub roll.
- Go for turkey, chicken, ham and roast beef. Avoid tuna, chicken and egg salads, salami, pepperoni and bologna.

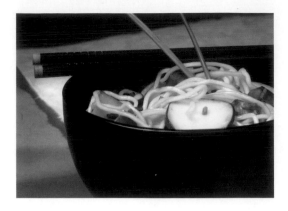

▷ Thai:

- Avoid anything in peanut sauce, peanuts or cashews.
- Avoid items that are crispy or deep-fried.
- Go for garlic, basil, ginger and brown sauces instead of curries.
- Have a stir-fry entrée prepared in broth rather than oil.
- Choose non-fried, rice-paper or lettuce-wrapped spring rolls.
- Pad Thai is a sure-fire diet buster.
- Satay is a smart start, but skip the peanut sauce.

Progress
JOURNAL

Journaling is an important weight management tool. Use this daily journal to get started and to track your ongoing progress.

Your Progress Journal

Don't underestimate the importance of a daily progress journal. This powerful tracking tool has helped countless dieters reach their weight-loss goals and maintain their healthy weight. Use it faithfully every day and it can do the same for you. Here's how it works:

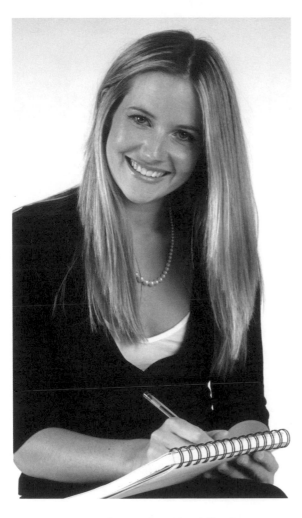

1 As you begin your new program, use your progress journal daily. It will help you to focus on your new program, evaluate your progress and gain a better understanding of your personal eating behaviors and activity level.

2 Every day you should write down what you eat, how much you exercise and how you are feeling about yourself and your goals. Don't forget to write down your successes and celebrate them!

3 Your progress journal provides a daily "snapshot" of your journey. As you progress, use your journal to help you better understand your personal challenges as well as your successes. Seeing how far you've come can give you the motivation you need to continue in times of weakness.

Use the **30-day journal** on the following pages as you begin your journey to a healthier new you! To continue tracking your progress beyond 30 days, photocopy the extra blank **measurement, fitness** and **journal log pages** in the back of this section.

About **You**

Your Name	
Your Current Weight	
Your Goal Weight	
Amount of Weight You Want To Lose	
BMI Goal	

What is the main reason you want to lose weight?

_____

_____

What type of exercise or sports do you like to participate in?

_____

_____

How will you celebrate when you reach your goal?

_____

_____

Who will you rely on when you need help along the way?

☐ **Family**   ☐ **Friends**   ☐ **Co-workers**   ☐ **Professional support**

Body **Measurements**

Tracking your body measurements can be a very effective assessment tool for monitoring your weight loss progress and updating your fitness program. A measurement history log can also be a very effective motivational tool.

When measuring, be sure to keep the tape measure against the skin so that it is not too snug or too loose. You should be able to fit one finger under the tape measure. Also, the accuracy of your measurements will depend on your ability to measure in the same spot each time. Descriptions on where to measure each body part have been provided to assist you in your accuracy.

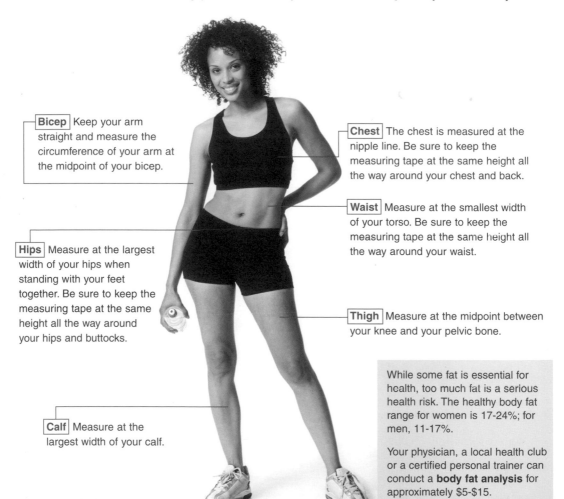

Bicep Keep your arm straight and measure the circumference of your arm at the midpoint of your bicep.

Hips Measure at the largest width of your hips when standing with your feet together. Be sure to keep the measuring tape at the same height all the way around your hips and buttocks.

Calf Measure at the largest width of your calf.

Chest The chest is measured at the nipple line. Be sure to keep the measuring tape at the same height all the way around your chest and back.

Waist Measure at the smallest width of your torso. Be sure to keep the measuring tape at the same height all the way around your waist.

Thigh Measure at the midpoint between your knee and your pelvic bone.

While some fat is essential for health, too much fat is a serious health risk. The healthy body fat range for women is 17-24%; for men, 11-17%.

Your physician, a local health club or a certified personal trainer can conduct a **body fat analysis** for approximately $5-$15.

Track Your Progress

Measurement Log

	Start Date	Day 15	Day 30
Date			
Weight (lbs.)			
Body Fat (%)			
Bicep (inches)			
Chest (inches)			
Waist (inches)			
Hips (inches)			
Thigh (inches)			
Calf (inches)			
Notes / Thoughts			

Daily Exercise Log

	Date	Time	Type of Exercise	Activity
Example	**April 12, 2006**	**8:00** (am)/ pm	☒ Cardio ☐ Strength	**Brisk walking**
		am / pm	☐ Cardio ☐ Strength	
		am / pm	☐ Cardio ☐ Strength	
		am / pm	☐ Cardio ☐ Strength	
		am / pm	☐ Cardio ☐ Strength	
		am / pm	☐ Cardio ☐ Strength	
		am / pm	☐ Cardio ☐ Strength	
		am / pm	☐ Cardio ☐ Strength	
		am / pm	☐ Cardio ☐ Strength	
		am / pm	☐ Cardio ☐ Strength	
		am / pm	☐ Cardio ☐ Strength	
		am / pm	☐ Cardio ☐ Strength	
		am / pm	☐ Cardio ☐ Strength	
		am / pm	☐ Cardio ☐ Strength	

Duration (Minutes)	Set / Reps	How do you feel?
20	/	I got started, but tired. More tomorrow!
	/	
	/	
	/	
	/	
	/	
	/	
	/	
	/	
	/	
	/	
	/	
	/	

Day 1

TIP OF THE DAY

High fiber diets will keep you healthier! Fiber fills you up, not out! High-fiber foods include whole grains and whole-grain breads and cereals, whole pieces of fruit and vegetables, legumes and salads.

▷ Daily Essentials

8-oz. Glasses of Water:
1 ☐ 2 ☐ 3 ☐ 4 ☐ 5 ☐ 6 ☐ 7 ☐ 8 ☐

Multivitamin Supplement: ☐

▷ Personal Goals, Thoughts & Notes

_____

_____

_____

_____

_____

_____

▷ Daily Meals

Breakfast _____

_____

Lunch _____

_____

Dinner _____

_____

Snack(s) _____

_____

TIP OF THE DAY	*Enjoy your food. Chew slowly; savor the mouth sensations, aromas and tastes. You'll find you're fuller and more satisfied when you take the time to savor your food and appreciate food's nutrition.*

▷ Daily Essentials

8-oz. Glasses of Water:
        1 ☐ 2 ☐ 3 ☐ 4 ☐ 5 ☐ 6 ☐ 7 ☐ 8 ☐

Multivitamin Supplement: ☐

▷ Personal Goals, Thoughts & Notes

_____

_____

_____

_____

_____

_____

▷ Daily Meals

Breakfast _____

_____

Lunch _____

_____

Dinner _____

_____

Snack(s) _____

_____

Day 3

All carbohydrates are not created equal. Complex carbohydrates are "whole" foods; they are your body's primary energy source. Enjoy whole grain breads and cereals, whole pieces of fruit and vegetables.

▷ Daily Essentials

8-oz. Glasses of Water: 1 ☐ 2 ☐ 3 ☐ 4 ☐ 5 ☐ 6 ☐ 7 ☐ 8 ☐

Multivitamin Supplement: ☐

▷ Personal Goals, Thoughts & Notes

_____

_____

_____

_____

_____

_____

▷ Daily Meals

Breakfast _____

_____

Lunch _____

_____

Dinner _____

_____

Snack(s) _____

_____

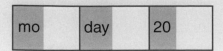

mo	day	20

TIP OF THE DAY | *Go fish! Tuna, salmon, haddock and sardines contain unsaturated omega-3 fatty acids, which may reduce the risk of heart disease and reduce inflammation from rheumatoid arthritis.*

▷ Daily Essentials

8-oz. Glasses of Water: 1 ☐ 2 ☐ 3 ☐ 4 ☐ 5 ☐ 6 ☐ 7 ☐ 8 ☐

Multivitamin Supplement: ☐

▷ Personal Goals, Thoughts & Notes

_____

_____

_____

_____

_____

_____

▷ Daily Meals

Breakfast _____

_____

Lunch _____

_____

Dinner _____

_____

Snack(s) _____

_____

Day 5

TIP OF THE DAY

Drink your milk. If you think nonfat is too "watery," make it creamier by stirring in one packet of nonfat dried milk. You'll improve the texture while increasing the protein, calcium, riboflavin and vitamins A and D.

▷ Daily Essentials

8-oz. Glasses of Water: 1 ☐ 2 ☐ 3 ☐ 4 ☐ 5 ☐ 6 ☐ 7 ☐ 8 ☐

Multivitamin Supplement: ☐

▷ Personal Goals, Thoughts & Notes

_____

_____

_____

_____

_____

_____

▷ Daily Meals

Breakfast _____

_____

Lunch _____

_____

Dinner _____

_____

Snack(s) _____

_____

Day 6

Walking is great exercise, but don't stroll. Walk briskly for the most aerobic benefit. Walking for 30 minutes at 2 mph burns 84 calories, compared with 156 calories burned walking 4 mph.

▷ Daily Essentials

8-oz. Glasses of Water: 1 ☐   2 ☐   3 ☐   4 ☐   5 ☐   6 ☐   7 ☐   8 ☐

Multivitamin Supplement: ☐

▷ Personal Goals, Thoughts & Notes

_____

_____

_____

_____

_____

_____

▷ Daily Meals

Breakfast _____

_____

Lunch _____

_____

Dinner _____

_____

Snack(s) _____

_____

Day 7

TIP OF THE DAY

Build some muscle. Muscle is more metabolically active than fat and helps you burn calories. If you can, begin a light weight training schedule. Always check with your doctor before beginning.

▷ Daily Essentials

8-oz. Glasses of Water: 1 ☐ 2 ☐ 3 ☐ 4 ☐ 5 ☐ 6 ☐ 7 ☐ 8 ☐

Multivitamin Supplement: ☐

▷ Personal Goals, Thoughts & Notes

_____

_____

_____

_____

_____

_____

▷ Daily Meals

Breakfast _____

_____

Lunch _____

_____

Dinner _____

_____

Snack(s) _____

_____

mo		day		20	

TIP OF THE DAY

Get your ZZZs! Adequate rest is an important part of the good health equation. Most adults need an average of 8 hours of sleep to perform quality work, handle everyday stress and feel good.

▷ Daily Essentials

8-oz. Glasses of Water: 1 ☐ 2 ☐ 3 ☐ 4 ☐ 5 ☐ 6 ☐ 7 ☐ 8 ☐

Multivitamin Supplement: ☐

▷ Personal Goals, Thoughts & Notes

_____

_____

_____

_____

_____

_____

▷ Daily Meals

Breakfast _____

_____

Lunch _____

_____

Dinner _____

_____

Snack(s) _____

_____

Day 9

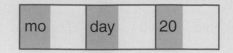

TIP OF THE DAY

Make every moment count. Sitting in a traffic jam? Use the time to isolate and tighten some muscle groups. Abdominals, gluteus maximus (rear end) and thighs ... hold for three seconds, relax and repeat several times.

▷ Daily Essentials

8-oz. Glasses of Water: 1 ☐ 2 ☐ 3 ☐ 4 ☐ 5 ☐ 6 ☐ 7 ☐ 8 ☐

Multivitamin Supplement: ☐

▷ Personal Goals, Thoughts & Notes

_____

_____

_____

_____

_____

_____

▷ Daily Meals

Breakfast _____

_____

Lunch _____

_____

Dinner _____

_____

Snack(s) _____

_____

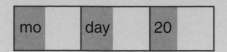

mo	day	20	

Day 10

TIP OF THE DAY

Black and green teas contain antioxidants that may prevent carcinogen development in the body. Tea drinkers may have lower blood pressure, cholesterol and heart disease rates. Both contain caffeine, so limit to two cups daily.

▷ Daily Essentials

8-oz. Glasses of Water: 1 ☐ 2 ☐ 3 ☐ 4 ☐ 5 ☐ 6 ☐ 7 ☐ 8 ☐

Multivitamin Supplement: ☐

▷ Personal Goals, Thoughts & Notes

_____

_____

_____

_____

_____

_____

▷ Daily Meals

Breakfast _____

_____

Lunch _____

_____

Dinner _____

_____

Snack(s) _____

_____

Day 11

TIP OF THE DAY

High blood cholesterol is a risk factor for heart disease. Avoid saturated fat and trans fat which is formed when liquid oil is made solid at room temperature in margarine and shortening. Olive, canola and peanut oils are the healthiest fats.

▷ Daily Essentials

8-oz. Glasses of Water: 1 ☐ 2 ☐ 3 ☐ 4 ☐ 5 ☐ 6 ☐ 7 ☐ 8 ☐

Multivitamin Supplement: ☐

▷ Personal Goals, Thoughts & Notes

_____

_____

_____

_____

_____

_____

▷ Daily Meals

Breakfast _____

_____

Lunch _____

_____

Dinner _____

_____

Snack(s) _____

_____

Keep food safe. Store leftovers in shallow containers and refrigerate or freeze within two hours of serving time to decrease unfriendly bacteria.

▷ Daily Essentials

8-oz. Glasses of Water: 1 ☐ 2 ☐ 3 ☐ 4 ☐ 5 ☐ 6 ☐ 7 ☐ 8 ☐

Multivitamin Supplement: ☐

▷ Personal Goals, Thoughts & Notes

_____

_____

_____

_____

_____

_____

▷ Daily Meals

Breakfast _____

_____

Lunch _____

_____

Dinner _____

_____

Snack(s) _____

_____

Day 13

TIP OF THE DAY

Think color! Eat a rainbow of nutrients ... red, orange, deep yellow and dark green leafy vegetables and fruits are great sources of carotenoids, important disease-fighting antioxidants.

▷ Daily Essentials

8-oz. Glasses of Water: 1 ☐ 2 ☐ 3 ☐ 4 ☐ 5 ☐ 6 ☐ 7 ☐ 8 ☐

Multivitamin Supplement: ☐

▷ Personal Goals, Thoughts & Notes

_____

_____

_____

_____

_____

_____

▷ Daily Meals

Breakfast _____

_____

Lunch _____

_____

Dinner _____

_____

Snack(s) _____

_____

mo		day		20	

TIP OF THE DAY

A cancer-prevention diet is one that is high in fiber, low in fat (especially animal fat), minimizes or excludes alcohol and includes generous portions of fresh fruits and vegetables.

▷ Daily Essentials

8-oz. Glasses of Water: 1 ☐ 2 ☐ 3 ☐ 4 ☐ 5 ☐ 6 ☐ 7 ☐ 8 ☐

Multivitamin Supplement: ☐

▷ Personal Goals, Thoughts & Notes

_____

_____

_____

_____

_____

_____

▷ Daily Meals

Breakfast _____

_____

Lunch _____

_____

Dinner _____

_____

Snack(s) _____

_____

Day 15

TIP OF THE DAY

Break your meals into "mini-meals" during the day to keep blood sugar levels stable and your motivation and energy levels high. You won't be hungry. This is a proven way to succeed on your weight-loss plan.

▷ Daily Essentials

8-oz. Glasses of Water: 1 ☐ 2 ☐ 3 ☐ 4 ☐ 5 ☐ 6 ☐ 7 ☐ 8 ☐

Multivitamin Supplement: ☐

▷ Personal Goals, Thoughts & Notes

_____

_____

_____

_____

_____

_____

▷ Daily Meals

Breakfast _____

_____

Lunch _____

_____

Dinner _____

_____

Snack(s) _____

_____

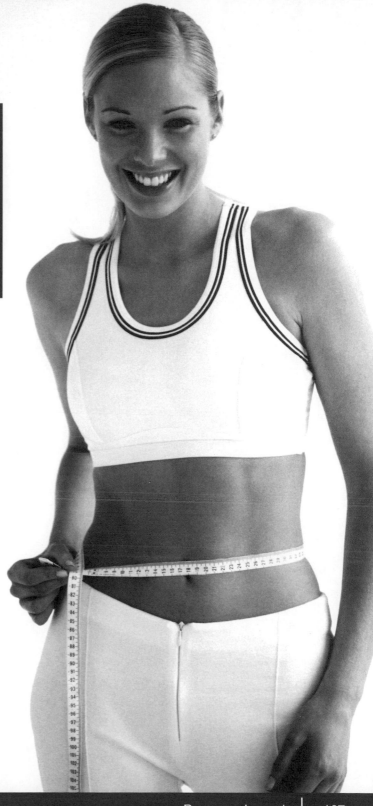

Reminder:

Today's the day to check your weight and measurements.

Day 16

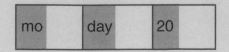
**TIP OF
THE DAY**

Eating healthy and losing excess weight will reduce your risk of heart disease. The relationship between cardiac disease, high blood pressure and Type 2 diabetes is well known.

▷ Daily Essentials

8-oz. Glasses of Water:
1 ☐ 2 ☐ 3 ☐ 4 ☐ 5 ☐ 6 ☐ 7 ☐ 8 ☐

Multivitamin Supplement: ☐

▷ Personal Goals, Thoughts & Notes

_____

_____

_____

_____

_____

_____

▷ Daily Meals

Breakfast _____

_____

Lunch _____

_____

Dinner _____

_____

Snack(s) _____

_____

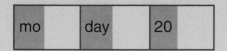
Day 17

Restaurant portion sizes are too large to eat in one sitting. Share an entree, order an appetizer as an entree with salad or soup, and ask for a "to-go" box as soon as your meal arrives.

▷ Daily Essentials

8-oz. Glasses of Water: ☐¹ ☐² ☐³ ☐⁴ ☐⁵ ☐⁶ ☐⁷ ☐⁸

Multivitamin Supplement: ☐

▷ Personal Goals, Thoughts & Notes

_____

_____

_____

_____

_____

_____

▷ Daily Meals

Breakfast _____

_____

Lunch _____

_____

Dinner _____

_____

Snack(s) _____

_____

Day 18

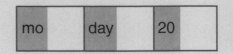
TIP OF THE DAY | *Season vegetables with herbs, spices or low-fat/sodium broth instead of fat or sauces. Tasty combinations include dill with carrots, rosemary on potatoes and vinegar on spinach.*

▷ Daily Essentials

8-oz. Glasses of Water: 1 ☐ 2 ☐ 3 ☐ 4 ☐ 5 ☐ 6 ☐ 7 ☐ 8 ☐

Multivitamin Supplement: ☐

▷ Personal Goals, Thoughts & Notes

_____

_____

_____

_____

_____

_____

▷ Daily Meals

Breakfast _____

_____

Lunch _____

_____

Dinner _____

_____

Snack(s) _____

_____

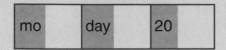

mo	day	20

TIP OF THE DAY | *Writing your goals down on paper is more inspirational than just thinking about them. Successful achievers create written contracts, set reasonable goals often and write them down.*

▷ Daily Essentials

8-oz. Glasses of Water:
1 ☐ 2 ☐ 3 ☐ 4 ☐ 5 ☐ 6 ☐ 7 ☐ 8 ☐

Multivitamin Supplement: ☐

▷ Personal Goals, Thoughts & Notes

_____
_____
_____
_____
_____
_____

▷ Daily Meals

Breakfast _____
_____

Lunch _____
_____

Dinner _____
_____

Snack(s) _____
_____

Day 20

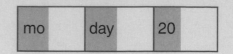

| TIP OF THE DAY | Be proactive about your health. If you have a family history of diabetes, heart disease or hypertension, it is especially important to eat right and maintain a healthy weight. |

▷ Daily Essentials

8-oz. Glasses of Water: 1 ☐ 2 ☐ 3 ☐ 4 ☐ 5 ☐ 6 ☐ 7 ☐ 8 ☐

Multivitamin Supplement: ☐

▷ Personal Goals, Thoughts & Notes

_____

_____

_____

_____

_____

_____

▷ Daily Meals

Breakfast _____

_____

Lunch _____

_____

Dinner _____

_____

Snack(s) _____

_____

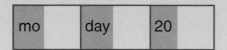
| TIP OF THE DAY | *It's not a "diet;" it's a "lifestyle change." You won't make all the changes overnight. It's one step at a time, one day at a time. With every successful day, you'll grow stronger.* |

▷ Daily Essentials

8-oz. Glasses of Water: 1 ☐ 2 ☐ 3 ☐ 4 ☐ 5 ☐ 6 ☐ 7 ☐ 8 ☐

Multivitamin Supplement: ☐

▷ Personal Goals, Thoughts & Notes

_____

_____

_____

_____

_____

_____

▷ Daily Meals

Breakfast _____

_____

Lunch _____

_____

Dinner _____

_____

Snack(s) _____

_____

Day 22

**TIP OF
THE DAY**

*Laughter is the best medicine. Laughing lowers blood pressure,
improves circulation and lessens pain. A good giggle induces the brain
to release endorphins.*

▷ Daily Essentials

8-oz. Glasses of Water:
1 ☐ 2 ☐ 3 ☐ 4 ☐ 5 ☐ 6 ☐ 7 ☐ 8 ☐

Multivitamin Supplement: ☐

▷ Personal Goals, Thoughts & Notes

_____

_____

_____

_____

_____

_____

▷ Daily Meals

Breakfast _____

_____

Lunch _____

_____

Dinner _____

_____

Snack(s) _____

_____

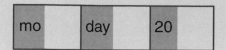

mo	day	20

TIP OF THE DAY	*Talk to yourself and remind yourself that you are your own best friend. The changes that you make for yourself are the most valuable changes imaginable. Pat yourself on the back daily ... you're the best!*

▷ Daily Essentials

8-oz. Glasses of Water: 1 ☐ 2 ☐ 3 ☐ 4 ☐ 5 ☐ 6 ☐ 7 ☐ 8 ☐

Multivitamin Supplement: ☐

▷ Personal Goals, Thoughts & Notes

_____

_____

_____

_____

_____

_____

▷ Daily Meals

Breakfast _____

_____

Lunch _____

_____

Dinner _____

_____

Snack(s) _____

_____

Day 24

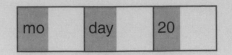
TIP OF THE DAY | *Your body needs at least eight glasses of water a day. It's easy when you take your water bottle with you wherever you go. Keep sipping at your desk and in the car.*

▷ Daily Essentials

8-oz. Glasses of Water:
1 ☐　2 ☐　3 ☐　4 ☐　5 ☐　6 ☐　7 ☐　8 ☐

Multivitamin Supplement: ☐

▷ Personal Goals, Thoughts & Notes

_____

_____

_____

_____

_____

_____

▷ Daily Meals

Breakfast _____

_____

Lunch _____

_____

Dinner _____

_____

Snack(s) _____

_____

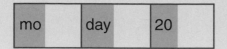
TIP OF THE DAY	*Choose a variety of foods to get all the different vitamins, minerals and phytochemicals you need to stay healthy. Don't eat the same thing every day. Variety promotes good health.*

▷ Daily Essentials

8-oz. Glasses of Water: 1 ☐   2 ☐   3 ☐   4 ☐   5 ☐   6 ☐   7 ☐   8 ☐

Multivitamin Supplement: ☐

▷ Personal Goals, Thoughts & Notes

_____

_____

_____

_____

_____

▷ Daily Meals

Breakfast _____

_____

Lunch _____

_____

Dinner _____

_____

Snack(s) _____

_____

Day 26

TIP OF THE DAY

There are no "bad" foods. Even chocolate has its place in a healthy diet. Enjoy low-fat chocolate with sugar-free hot chocolate or nonfat chocolate pudding as a serving of milk in your healthy meal plan.

▷ **Daily Essentials**

8-oz. Glasses of Water: 1 ☐   2 ☐   3 ☐   4 ☐   5 ☐   6 ☐   7 ☐   8 ☐

Multivitamin Supplement: ☐

▷ **Personal Goals, Thoughts & Notes**

_____

_____

_____

_____

_____

_____

▷ **Daily Meals**

Breakfast _____

_____

Lunch _____

_____

Dinner _____

_____

Snack(s) _____

_____

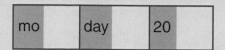

TIP OF THE DAY

You are what you think you are, so think good thoughts. By focusing on your positive characteristics, you'll build the strength to keep making changes for the better.

▷ Daily Essentials

8-oz. Glasses of Water: 1 ☐ 2 ☐ 3 ☐ 4 ☐ 5 ☐ 6 ☐ 7 ☐ 8 ☐

Multivitamin Supplement: ☐

▷ Personal Goals, Thoughts & Notes

_____

_____

_____

_____

_____

_____

▷ Daily Meals

Breakfast _____

_____

Lunch _____

_____

Dinner _____

_____

Snack(s) _____

_____

Day 28

TIP OF THE DAY | *Start your day with a healthy breakfast. It's the easiest meal to get good fiber with a high-fiber cereal, low-fat or nonfat milk and whole fruit.*

▷ Daily Essentials

8-oz. Glasses of Water: 1 ☐ 2 ☐ 3 ☐ 4 ☐ 5 ☐ 6 ☐ 7 ☐ 8 ☐

Multivitamin Supplement: ☐

▷ Personal Goals, Thoughts & Notes

_____

_____

_____

_____

_____

_____

▷ Daily Meals

Breakfast _____

_____

Lunch _____

_____

Dinner _____

_____

Snack(s) _____

_____

Day 29

| TIP OF THE DAY | *Exercise makes you feel good. It helps reduce your risk of heart disease and stroke by strengthening the heart muscle, lowering blood pressure and boosting "good" HDL cholesterol.* |

▷ Daily Essentials

8-oz. Glasses of Water: 1 ☐ 2 ☐ 3 ☐ 4 ☐ 5 ☐ 6 ☐ 7 ☐ 8 ☐

Multivitamin Supplement: ☐

▷ Personal Goals, Thoughts & Notes

_____

_____

_____

_____

_____

_____

▷ Daily Meals

Breakfast _____

_____

Lunch _____

_____

Dinner _____

_____

Snack(s) _____

_____

Day 30

TIP OF THE DAY

Low-calorie diets don't work. Why put yourself through torture and slow your metabolism? Slow and steady weight loss of two pounds per week is a surefire way to succeed.

▷ **Daily Essentials**

8-oz. Glasses of Water: 1 ☐   2 ☐   3 ☐   4 ☐   5 ☐   6 ☐   7 ☐   8 ☐

Multivitamin Supplement: ☐

▷ **Personal Goals, Thoughts & Notes**

_____

_____

_____

_____

_____

_____

▷ **Daily Meals**

Breakfast _____

_____

Lunch _____

_____

Dinner _____

_____

Snack(s) _____

_____

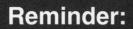

Reminder:

Today's the day to check your weight and measurements.

Extra Log Pages

Measurement Log (Every 15 Days)

Date			
Weight (lbs.)			
Body Fat (%)			
Bicep (inches)			
Chest (inches)			
Waist (inches)			
Hips (inches)			
Thigh (inches)			
Calf (inches)			
Notes / Thoughts			

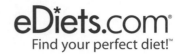

Measurement Log (Every 15 Days)

Date			
Weight (lbs.)			
Body Fat (%)			
Bicep (inches)			
Chest (inches)			
Waist (inches)			
Hips (inches)			
Thigh (inches)			
Calf (inches)			
Notes / Thoughts			

Daily Exercise Log

Date	Time	Type of Exercise	Activity
	am / pm	☐ Cardio ☐ Strength	
	am / pm	☐ Cardio ☐ Strength	
	am / pm	☐ Cardio ☐ Strength	
	am / pm	☐ Cardio ☐ Strength	
	am / pm	☐ Cardio ☐ Strength	
	am / pm	☐ Cardio ☐ Strength	
	am / pm	☐ Cardio ☐ Strength	
	am / pm	☐ Cardio ☐ Strength	
	am / pm	☐ Cardio ☐ Strength	
	am / pm	☐ Cardio ☐ Strength	
	am / pm	☐ Cardio ☐ Strength	
	am / pm	☐ Cardio ☐ Strength	
	am / pm	☐ Cardio ☐ Strength	
	am / pm	☐ Cardio ☐ Strength	

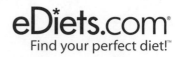

Duration (Minutes)	Set / Reps	How do you feel?
	/	
	/	
	/	
	/	
	/	
	/	
	/	
	/	
	/	
	/	
	/	
	/	
	/	
	/	

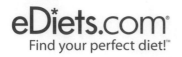

| Day: | | mo | | day | | 20 | |

▷ Daily Essentials

8-oz. Glasses of Water: 1 ☐ 2 ☐ 3 ☐ 4 ☐ 5 ☐ 6 ☐ 7 ☐ 8 ☐

Multivitamin Supplement: ☐

▷ Personal Goals, Thoughts & Notes

_____

_____

_____

_____

_____

_____

▷ Daily Meals

Breakfast _____

_____

Lunch _____

_____

Dinner _____

_____

Snack(s) _____

_____

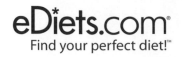

Day:		mo		day		20	

▷ Daily Essentials

8-oz. Glasses of Water:
       1   2   3   4   5   6   7   8
       ☐   ☐   ☐   ☐   ☐   ☐   ☐   ☐

Multivitamin Supplement: ☐

▷ Personal Goals, Thoughts & Notes

_____

_____

_____

_____

_____

_____

_____

▷ Daily Meals

Breakfast _____

_____

Lunch _____

_____

Dinner _____

_____

Snack(s) _____

_____

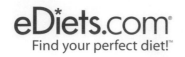

| Day: | | mo | | day | | 20 | |

▷ Daily Essentials

8-oz. Glasses of Water: 1 ☐ 2 ☐ 3 ☐ 4 ☐ 5 ☐ 6 ☐ 7 ☐ 8 ☐

Multivitamin Supplement: ☐

▷ Personal Goals, Thoughts & Notes

_____

_____

_____

_____

_____

_____

_____

▷ Daily Meals

Breakfast _____

_____

Lunch _____

_____

Dinner _____

_____

Snack(s) _____

_____

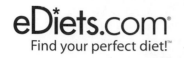
Find your perfect diet!™

| Day: | | mo | | day | | 20 | |

▷ Daily Essentials

8-oz. Glasses of Water:　1 ☐　2 ☐　3 ☐　4 ☐　5 ☐　6 ☐　7 ☐　8 ☐

Multivitamin Supplement: ☐

▷ Personal Goals, Thoughts & Notes

_____

_____

_____

_____

_____

_____

▷ Daily Meals

Breakfast _____

_____

Lunch _____

_____

Dinner _____

_____

Snack(s) _____

_____

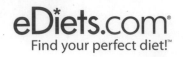
eDiets.com®
Find your perfect diet!™

| Day: | | mo | | day | | 20 | |

▷ Daily Essentials

8-oz. Glasses of Water:
1 ☐ 2 ☐ 3 ☐ 4 ☐ 5 ☐ 6 ☐ 7 ☐ 8 ☐

Multivitamin Supplement: ☐

▷ Personal Goals, Thoughts & Notes

_____

_____

_____

_____

_____

_____

_____

▷ Daily Meals

Breakfast _____

_____

Lunch _____

_____

Dinner _____

_____

Snack(s) _____

_____